Practical Assessment and Treatment of the Patient with Headaches in the Emergency Department and Urgent Care Clinic

Dawn A. Marcus · Philip A. Bain

Practical Assessment and Treatment of the Patient with Headaches in the Emergency Department and Urgent Care Clinic

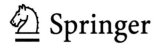 Springer

Dawn A. Marcus, MD
Professor
Department of Anesthesiology
University of Pittsburgh
Pittsburgh, PA, USA
dawn.a.marcus@gmail.com

Philip A. Bain, MD
Dean Health Systems
Madison, WI, USA
philip.bain@deancare.com

Please note that additional material for this book can be downloaded from http://extras.springer.com

ISBN 978-1-4614-0001-1   e-ISBN 978-1-4614-0002-8
DOI 10.1007/978-1-4614-0002-8
Springer New York Dordrecht Heidelberg London

Library of Congress Control Number: 2011931278

Printed on acid-free paper

Springer is part of Springer Science+Business Media (www.springer.com)

Preface

Headache is a nearly universal symptom. Migraine, one of the most common types of headache, affects 28 million Americans, including one in six adult women. In 2006, headache accounted for nearly 3% of all emergency department (ED) visits, resulting in almost 3.4 million visits. It was the sixth most common reason for ED visits that year.

Currently, there are no widely used guidelines for the treatment of patients with headache in the ED or Urgent Care Clinic. In one study, 35 drugs, alone or in combination, were used to treat migraine, with narcotics the most commonly selected therapy. Lack of specific training in managing headache patients and the need to efficiently move patients through a busy ED can result in significant frustration for the ED staff confronted with the patient complaining of an acute headache.

During our research for this book, we surveyed practicing ED doctors and asked what they found most frustrating about headache patients and what would most help them improve their care of ED patients complaining of headache. The answers to these surveys provided consistent themes:

- ED doctors are frustrated with patients with chronic headache who come to the ED requesting narcotic therapy.
- ED doctors are concerned about missing the diagnosis of serious, life-threatening headaches.
- ED doctors would like to improve communication with primary care physicians and neurologists treating headache patients as outpatients.
- Practical strategies are needed for understanding what outpatient providers prefer their patients receive when treated in the ED for chronic headache. Mechanisms are also needed to provide feedback to outpatient clinicians.
- ED doctors would like practical advice about using a wide variety of effective headache treatment options, including procedures like occipital nerve blocks and nondrug therapies.
- ED doctors would like to help patients get appropriate timely outpatient follow-up and help patients understand that a definitive diagnosis and care should be provided through post-ED follow-up care.

- ED doctors would like to be able to significantly decrease unnecessary return visits for headache treatment.

We have tried to address each of these concerns in this book. While the convention throughout the book is to refer to ED patients, ED care, etc., these same principles may also be applied to headache patients seen in Urgent Care Clinics.

Practical Assessment and Treatment of the Patient with Headaches in the Emergency Department and Urgent Care Clinic was designed with the practicing ED provider in mind. This book draws upon both clinical expertise and an extensive published literature to provide clinicians with recommendations for effective and efficient care of the ED headache patient. Co-authored by Drs. Dawn A. Marcus and Philip A. Bain, this book provides information from both headache specialty research as well as experience in primary care. Dr. Dawn Marcus is a neurologist, headache specialist, and professor at the University of Pittsburgh. Dr. Philip Bain is a general internist in a large multispecialty group in Madison, WI, who has a longstanding interest in treatment of headache disorders at the primary care level. Together, Drs. Marcus and Bain draw on over 40 years of clinical experience caring for patients with headache. Drs. Marcus and Bain have previously collaborated in writing two other practical books on managing headache: *Effective Migraine Treatment in Pregnant and Lactating Women* and *The Woman's Migraine Toolkit. Managing Headaches from Puberty to Menopause.*

Practical Assessment and Treatment of the Patient with Headaches in the Emergency Department and Urgent Care Clinic uses easy-to-understand figures, charts, and algorithms to help make this book a practical resource, with downloadable tools (including patient handouts) available at the Publisher's web site at http://extras.springer.com. Photographs showing techniques for diagnostic as well as headache-relieving procedures and commonly encountered imaging abnormalities are also included. Two unique features of this book are the focus on post-ED followup care to reduce unnecessary repeat visits for the same headache and a risk management chapter that addresses issues such as how to deal with inappropriate demands for opioid pain killers, common cognitive errors, and how to avoid common legal pitfalls in the ED. *Practical Assessment and Treatment of the Patient with Headaches in the Emergency Department and Urgent Care Clinic* addresses the full spectrum of headaches seen in the ED, including chronic migraine, traumatic headaches, secondary headaches, and headaches occurring in pediatric, obstetric, and older adult patients.

The authors welcome your comments about this book, your experiences, and information on other proven methods that would be helpful for future editions. Comments can be left at http://www.dawnmarcusmd.com.

Pittsburgh, PA   Dawn A. Marcus
Madison, WI   Philip A. Bain

Acknowledgments

The authors would like to thank the following colleagues for their valuable comments and review of the materials contained in this book: Benjamin Friedman, MD, Merle Diamond, MD, Tim Hill, MD, Krishna Prasad, MD, Kyle Martin, MD, Tom Woodward, MD, Dave Gronski, MD, Brian Reeder, MD, A. David Rothner, MD, and Steve Linder, MD.

Gratitude is also extended to attorneys John Walsh, JD, Barrett J. Corneille, JD, and J. Michael Riley, JD for their insightful comments regarding legal issues involving patients with headaches seen in the emergency department. Also, Jane Crandall was very helpful in collating many of the legal related articles for this book.

Finally, we would like to acknowledge and thank David Shearer, MD, Michelle Mueller, and Kathy Miller for their help in demonstrating and photographing helpful procedures referenced in this book. We would additionally like to thank Rhea Marcus and Cheryl Noethiger for acting as models. We are also indebted to Clayton A. Wiley, MD, PhD, Rock Heyman, MD, and The Migraine Trust for the case histories and images they provided.

Contents

Chapter 1
Overview of Headache in the Emergency Department

Key Chapter Points

- About 2–3% of all ED visits are for headache.
- Migraine is the #1 diagnosis for nontraumatic headache seen in the emergency department, accounting for 40–60% of all nontraumatic, emergency department headaches.
- While migraine sufferers usually obtain routine headache care with outpatient providers, ED treatment is generally sought when pain becomes unbearable, patient's current headache regimen is not effective, or a patient's primary headache provider is unavailable.
- ED visits are expensive and often very frustrating for staff and patients.
- Common errors of ED headache assessment include focusing on identifying a specific primary headache diagnosis rather than distinguishing primary from secondary headaches, misunderstanding the role of hypertension, failing to identify unreported trauma, and using treatment response to confirm a diagnosis.

Keywords Acute migraine • Cost • Nausea • Nontraumatic

Box 1.1 Case Presentation

Janice is a 37-year-old mother who presents to the emergency department (ED) with a chief complaint of severe headache and nausea. She has had migraines since she was in college. Her headaches are usually well managed at home with over-the-counter analgesics and a nap. Her current headache began the previous evening and failed to respond to her usual treatments. After sending her boys to school this morning, she came to the ED. Janice has been in a crowded waiting room for the last 2 h, holding a damp wash cloth over her eyes, moaning, and occasionally dry heaving into an emesis basin

(continued)

D.A. Marcus and P.A. Bain, *Practical Assessment and Treatment of the Patient with Headaches in the Emergency Department and Urgent Care Clinic*, DOI 10.1007/978-1-4614-0002-8_1, © Springer Science+Business Media, LLC 2011

Box 1.1 (continued)

she brought with her. "My headaches usually aren't this bad and my doctor's office doesn't open until 9, so I thought I'd just stop in the emergency room and get my headache taken care of right away. If I could just lie down in a dark quiet room, I'd feel so much better, but the nurse said I have to wait until they're less busy to take care of me. Sitting here under these fluorescent lights with people yelling and babies crying has just made everything even worse! I asked the nurse if they could just give me a strong pain killer that I could take home with me. She looked at me like I was a junkie or something! I'm sure the nurse is hoping I'll give up and leave, but I'm afraid if I leave now, I'll just end up having to wait even longer at my doctor's office."

In the ED, headache patients may be triaged to lower priority service, with more expedient care provided to patients with chest pain, severe infections, or trauma. Headache patients like Janice often become frustrated, as waiting in a busy, bright, loud ED can aggravate symptoms for many patients with severe headache. ED providers may be equally frustrated with visits from patients reporting chronic headaches, concerned that some of these patients may be malingering and drug seeking.

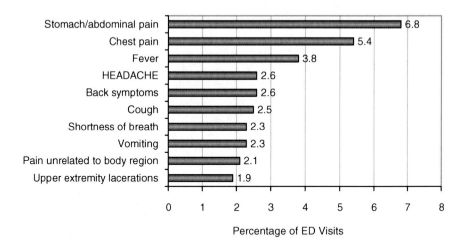

Fig. 1.1 Reasons for ED visits in the USA (based on [1] and reproduced with permission from Marcus DA and Bain PA. *Effective migraine treatment in pregnant and lactating women*. Humana Press 2009)

Headache is one of the most common symptoms resulting in emergency or urgent care treatment. Using national statistics data about emergency service use, headache accounted for 2.6% of all emergency visits, making headache the fourth most common reason for visiting an emergency department (ED), tied with back symptoms (Fig. 1.1) [1]. On average, six headache patients visit an ED every minute in the USA [2].

Although headache is frequently seen in the ED, headache is not an area of major focus during ED training. For example, disease area categories comprising the greatest weight on the American Board of Emergency Medicine's initial certification examination are trauma (11%) and cardiovascular (10%), abdominal and gastrointestinal (9%), and thoracic–respiratory disorders (8%) [3]. Categories that might contain headache include head, ear, eye, nose, and throat disorders (5% of the examination) and nervous system disorders (5%). Limited formal headache training and lack of available standardized or evidence-based management protocols for managing urgent headache complaints can make ED staff uncomfortable caring for headache patients. Furthermore, analgesics that offer only modest efficacy in primary headache, such as narcotics, are often routinely used for ED headache treatment, with limited benefit. These patients may return to the ED requesting additional care for persistent or recurrent headache, leading to a cycle of inappropriate, repeated ED visits for headache management and concerns about drug-seeking behavior.

Understanding the issues commonly seen in headache patients presenting to the ED and developing assessment and treatment strategies to expedite effective care can improve treatment outcomes for ED visits for headache. Satisfaction of both providers and patients may also improve by adopting streamlining strategies based on understanding which headache disorders most commonly present to the ED, why patients choose ED care, and what errors commonly confound ED headache management.

Most Non-traumatic Headaches in the ED Are Primary Headaches

Headaches can be divided into primary and secondary headaches. *Secondary* headaches can be directly attributed to underlying disease, pathology, or trauma, while *primary* headaches are not caused by another identifiable disease or medical condition.

> ***Pearl for the practitioner:***
> Primary headaches are those headaches, like migraine and tension-type headache, that are not attributed to other medical conditions. Secondary headaches are headaches directly caused by other underlying conditions or injury.

The second edition of the International Headache Classification ICHD-II diagnostic criteria lists 47 unique primary headaches [4]. The most common primary headaches are migraine and tension-type headaches (Table 1.1). Several primary headaches are short-lived and infrequently seen in the ED; typical durations of these relatively short-duration headaches are 60–90 min for cluster headaches, 2–30 min for paroxysmal hemicrania, and seconds to minutes for short-lasting unilateral neuralgiform headache attacks with conjunctival injection and tearing (SUNCT syndrome) and short-lasting unilateral neuralgiform headache attacks with cranial autonomic symptoms (SUNA syndrome).

Table 1.1 Primary headache disorders (ICHD-II criteria)

Primary headache disorder	Description	Attack frequency
Very short duration headaches (lasting seconds to minutes)		
Short-lasting unilateral neuralgiform headache attacks with conjunctival injection and tearing (SUNCT syndrome)	Unilateral head pain with marked, eye redness and tearing on the same side of the head pain	Frequent attacks throughout the day
Short-lasting unilateral neuralgiform headache attacks with cranial autonomic symptoms (SUNA syndrome)	SUNCT-like attacks that have either conjunctival injection OR tearing but not both OR other autonomic symptoms (lacrimation, rhinorrhea, eyelid edema)	Frequent attacks throughout the day
Stabbing headache (ice pick headache, jabs and jolts)	Localized stabs of pain in the head, typically affecting the periorbital, temporal, or parietal regions	Episodes recur irregularly
Cough headache	Diffuse or nondescript head pain	Head pain precipitated by cough, straining, or Valsalva maneuver
Thunderclap headache	Severe head pain with peak intensity in <1 min	Infrequently recurs
Short-lasting headaches (duration minutes to 3 h)		
Cluster headache	Excruciating, generally unilateral periorbital pain. Patient often hits head, showers, paces, or smokes during these 30–120 min intense attacks. Autonomic symptoms (lacrimation, rhinorrhea, etc.) typically occur but are unnoticed by patients due to intensity of pain. Alcohol can trigger attacks during a cluster period	Attacks often occur each night (often about 1 h after falling asleep) and occur in groups or clusters. Patients can have 1–4 attacks daily during the typical 6–8 week cluster. More common in the spring and fall
Paroxysmal hemicrania	Excruciating, unilateral periorbital or temple pain lasting for 2–30 min. Autonomic symptoms (lacrimation, rhinorrhea, etc.) typically occur	Typically >5 attacks daily
Exertional headache (weight lifters' headache)	Throbbing head pain lasting minutes to 2 days	Head pain triggered by exercise, especially during hot weather or at high altitudes

Headache type		
Headache associated with sexual activity (orgasmic headache)	Pain is usually mild and bilateral as sexual excitement intensifies, with pain peaking with orgasm or in the period immediately preceding orgasm	Triggered by sexual activity. Secondary headaches must be ruled out before attributing this type of headache to primary headache
Hypnic headache (alarm clock headache)	Diffuse, bilateral pain in adults >50 years old	Occurs at night, typically waking patient from sleep. Often occurs between 1 and 3 a.m.
Moderate–long duration headaches (typically 4 h–days)		
Migraine	Intermittent, disabling, sick headache typically lasting 4–72 h (usually 8–24 h) and associated with sensitivity to noises, lights, odors, and other stimulation. Pain is often located on one side of the head and throbbing. Patients prefer dark, quiet solitude during attacks. Transient neurological symptoms or aura (often visual disturbance) occur before or at the beginning of migraine attacks for 15–20%	Recurring, discrete headache episodes, often triggered by menses, stress, sleep deprivation, and fasting
Tension-type headache (muscle contraction headache, stress headache, "regular" headache)	Intermittent or constant, nondisabling headache. Pain is generally mild and often a pressure or squeezing sensation on both sides of the head. Daily routine is generally not affected by these headaches. Nausea/vomiting and light/sound sensitivity are generally absent	Recurring headache episodes or prolonged headache. Often triggered by stress and muscle overuse. Rarely disabling enough to trigger ED visit
Hemicrania continua	Unilateral pain always affecting the same side of the head and associated with unilateral autonomic features (e.g., lacrimation and rhinorrhea)	Continuous or very prolonged pain
New daily persistent headache (chronic headache)	Nondisabling, bilateral pressure pain	Daily, continuous head pain

Primary headaches are diagnosed in patients for whom secondary headaches have been ruled out as many secondary features share characteristics of most primary headaches

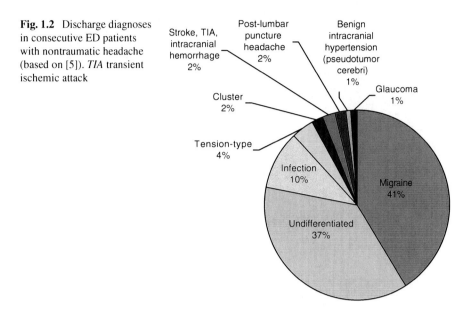

Fig. 1.2 Discharge diagnoses in consecutive ED patients with nontraumatic headache (based on [5]). *TIA* transient ischemic attack

In most cases, nontraumatic head pain seen in the ED is caused by benign, primary, recurring headaches. In a prospective, 11-month, observational survey, discharge diagnoses were analyzed for all ED patients presenting with a chief complaint of nontraumatic headache [5]. Migraine was the most common diagnosis, with only 16% of headaches assigned a secondary headache diagnosis (Fig. 1.2).

Similarly, data from the National Hospital Ambulatory Medical Care Survey reported 2.1 million ED visits annually for nontraumatic headache, accounting for 2.2% of all ED visits [6]. In this survey, migraine was again the most common single diagnosis, affecting two in every three patients treated in the ED for nontraumatic headache (63.5%). The next most common diagnoses were tension-type headache (3.4%), viral syndrome (2.4%), and anxiety/psychiatric diagnosis (1.1%). Twenty percent of headaches were diagnosed as "other benign conditions," including hypertension and infectious conditions affecting the ears, sinuses, or throat, gastroenteritis, or periapical (tooth) abscess. Pathological diagnoses (including meningitis, encephalitis, stroke, hemorrhage, aneurysm, glaucoma, benign intracranial hypertension, giant cell/ temporal arteritis, or hypertensive encephalopathy) were assigned to only 2% of headaches among all patients seen for nontraumatic headache. A pathological diagnosis

---

Pearl for the practitioner:
Migraine is the single most common cause of nontraumatic headache in patients seen in the ED:

- Up to 60% of patients seen in the ED for nontraumatic headache will have migraine.
- Rare but important secondary headaches are more common in middle and older aged adults, especially in patients over age 75. These will be covered in detail in Chap. 3.

was most common in middle and older aged adults, accounting for 6% of nontraumatic headaches in patients ≥50 years old and 11% in those ≥75 years old. The evaluation for possible secondary headaches is detailed in Chap. 3.

Why Do Headache Patients Come to the ED?

The ED is generally not the ideal environment for managing headaches. Most patients seeking ED treatment for nontraumatic head pain have primary headaches, especially migraine. Migraine sufferers usually prefer dark, quiet, comforting solitude during severe headaches – the exact opposite of most EDs. Also, patients with acute headaches presenting to the ED may be viewed by ED personnel as potential drug seekers or patients seeking inappropriate ED care for nonemergent conditions. Headache experts agree that chronic headaches are best managed in outpatient facilities rather than the ED. For a variety of reasons, however, many patients, like Janice, will at least occasionally seek out ED treatment.

Although primary headaches constitute the bulk of ED visits for nontraumatic headache, most patients with severe headache are managed outside of an emergency setting. A survey of 13,451 adults with severe headache found that only 6% had visited an ED during the preceding year, with half of these using the ED on only a single occasion [7]. Frequent ED use occurred for only 1% of the sample, although this minority of patients constituted 51% of all ED headache visits. Understanding why patients repeatedly seek ED treatment and devising strategies to facilitate more appropriate outpatient management can reduce episodes of frequent, often inappropriate use of the ED for primary headache management.

> **Pearl for the practitioner:**
> Most patients with severe headache obtain care outside of the ED. Over half of all ED visits for severe, nontraumatic headache are made by a small minority of patients who repeatedly seek headache care in the ED. Strategies need to be developed to minimize inappropriate return visits for this group of patients.

ED care is also an expensive way to manage chronic headaches. A review of ED visits for migraine in 2005 reported that the average per-patient cost for an ED visit for migraine was $1,799 [8]. This total did not include additional charges for transportation to the ED (with 24% of patients having arrived at the ED via ambulance) or radiologist fees for interpreting neuroimaging studies, which had been performed in 22% of patients.

If the ED is not very conducive to headache management and is so costly, then why is headache such a common chief complaint for ED visits? To understand why headache patients come to the ED, people with severe headache participating in the American Migraine Prevalence and Prevention study were asked about ED use [7]. Among the 859 individuals surveyed who had visited an ED at least once during the previous year, unbearable pain and inability to contact an outpatient provider were

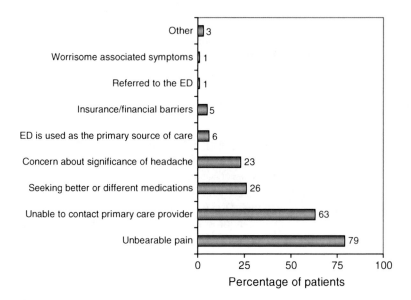

Fig. 1.3 Reasons for headache patients sought headache care in the ED during the previous year (based on [7]). Patients were allowed to endorse >1 reason

the most common reasons cited for seeking headache care in the ED (Fig. 1.3). These data highlight a tremendous opportunity. Many of these patients might more appropriately seek headache management in an outpatient, primary care practice if the opportunity were available. Also, these data suggest that, by appropriately diagnosing patients, initiating effective treatment, and arranging post-ED follow-up care, future unnecessary ED visits for recurring headaches can be minimized. A well thought out headache strategy can lead to more satisfied patients and providers as well as more cost-effective care.

> **Pearl for the practitioner:**
> Migraine sufferers who present to the ED for headache usually do so because of unbearable pain and an inability to obtain care from their primary care provider or other headache-interested provider. A coordinated plan of care and ongoing relationship with a headache-interested provider can dramatically reduce ED visits for headache.

ED Headache Treatment is Often Unsatisfactory for Both Patients and ED Staff

Many patients fail to achieve a satisfactory outcome when receiving ED management for nontraumatic headaches. A survey of 219 patients seen in the ED for acute nontraumatic headache reported insufficient treatment and persistent headache for a substantial number of surveyed patients [9]. Two-thirds of the patients in this sample were diagnosed with migraine. During their ED visit, two-thirds of the patients were treated with medications, most commonly neuroleptics or opioids, while one-third received neither medications nor intravenous rehydration. Only 22% were pain-free at discharge, with moderate to severe headache remaining in 35%. Furthermore, diaries completed during the 24-h after discharge showed that headache returned for 64% of patients.

> **Pearl for the practitioner:**
> Studies have shown that one in three patients presenting to the ED with acute headache will continue to report moderate or severe headache upon ED discharge. Headache will recur in two of three patients during the first day after ED discharge.

ED staff are also often dissatisfied with headache management. Working in an ED is difficult and can be frustrating. Data collected in 2004 reported that, while 65% of emergency physicians endorsed high career satisfaction, 33% reported that burnout was a significant problem [10]. A subsequent survey of a random sample from the American College of Emergency Physicians about career satisfaction and burnout published in 2009 likewise identified that 32% of doctors endorsed high levels of career burnout [11]. Burnout was significantly related to anxiety caused by diagnostic uncertainty and concern about potentially bad patient outcomes. Concerns about undiagnosed secondary headaches, dealing with drug-seeking behavior, and repeat visits by patients with persistent headache can add to the frustration of ED staff when caring for headache patients.

Some of the conflicts encountered in the ED may occur because patients and ED staff have different definitions of when patients should seek ED care. In an interesting study, adults shopping in supermarkets and malls were recruited for a survey, which was also completed by healthcare providers [12]. Responses were obtained from 1,018 lay people and 126 ED healthcare workers (Table 1.2). A significant difference of opinion identified between lay persons and ED workers was the feeling by lay persons (not shared by any ED workers) that having a medical problem outside of usual business hours represented a reason to seek ED treatment. Also, lay persons were asked to identify which of 30 chief complaints would require ED care. Lay persons and ED workers differed in their perceptions that severe headache would be considered an emergency condition. Interestingly, while 91% of ED workers identified severe headache as an emergency problem, only 58% of lay persons did so.

> **Pearl for the practitioner:**
> A substantial number of patients consider the occurrence of medical problems after hours to constitute an appropriate reason to seek ED care.

Table 1.2 Lay people and ED workers were asked to choose the best definition of an emergency medical condition (based on [12])

Definition of an emergency medical condition	Lay persons (%)	ED workers (%)
A condition that may result in death or permanent disability or cause severe pain	49	72
A condition that may result in death or permanent disability, cause severe pain, or prevent work	3	0
A condition that may result in death or permanent disability or cause severe pain OR any condition needing attention outside of normal business hours	17	0
Any condition at any time as determined by the patient	32	27

Common Traps Leading to Assessment Errors in Headache Care in the ED

Dr. Swadron from the ED at the University of Southern California recently published an article describing frequent pitfalls of headache management in the ED [13]. Commonly encountered pitfalls included problems with the assessment of headache patients (detailed below), misinterpretation of test results when ruling out secondary headaches, reliance on treatment options with a lower likelihood of good analgesic response (e.g., opioids), and failing to establish post-ED headache follow-up, especially for patients with primary headaches that would likely be expected to recur. Several of the most common traps identified as causes for error are detailed below.

Trap 1. Trying to Determine a Specific Primary Headache Diagnosis

The ICHD-II standard classifies headaches in a 149-page comprehensive reference with descriptions and diagnostic criteria for over 200 headache disorders, including over 40 individual primary headache diagnoses [4]. While providing an important anchor for headache research, this standard is too cumbersome and impractical for many busy clinical settings, especially the ED. The main focus of the ED headache assessment should be to distinguish patients with benign primary headaches from those with secondary headaches for which the condition causing the headache requires specific treatment.

In general, many of the same treatment principles and medications can be successfully utilized in patients with a variety of primary headaches. For example, both migraine and tension-type headaches share common clinical features and show similarly good response to medications, including drugs traditionally listed as "migraine-specific" therapies, such as the triptans [14]. In an interesting study, 480 patients with a primary ED complaint of nontraumatic headache not associated with altered mental status or malignancy were evaluated with a 100-item, standardized headache assessment interview based on ICHD-II criteria [15]. A total of 309 patients were determined to have a primary headache disorder (64%). Among these, the most common diagnoses were migraine ($N = 186$, 60%) and unclassified headache ($N = 77$, 25%). This study revealed that a specific headache diagnosis could not be identified for a substantial number of patients presenting to the ED with a primary headache disorder. These data underscore that it is more productive to rule out secondary headaches than to focus on which specific type of primary headache is present.

> **Pearl for the practitioner:**
> One in four patients determined to have a primary headache in the ED will be discharged without a specific headache diagnosis. Distinguishing primary from secondary headache is more important in the ED than establishing a specific primary headache diagnosis.

Trap 2. Making Diagnoses Contingent on Treatment Response

Primary headaches are diagnosed by clinical features and the absence of abnormalities on examination. Primary headaches cannot be diagnosed by treatment response. Patients experiencing headache relief from analgesics or the so-called migraine-specific medications may have migraine, but they may also have another primary headache or even secondary headaches. For example, two studies treating ED patients with sumatriptan, droperidol, or analgesics showed similar good efficacy in patients with migraine, tension-type headache, and primary headaches not meeting full criteria for a diagnosis of migraine [16, 17]. Triptans also can acutely relieve less common primary headaches, like cluster headaches [18]. Furthermore, sumatriptan has been reported to successfully relieve headaches due to a wide range of serious causes, including meningitis [19], subarachnoid hemorrhage [20, 21], carotid dissection [22], head and neck cancer [23], and others. Low pressure headaches, such as postdural puncture or spinal headaches, may also respond to treatment with the "migraine-specific" treatments, ergotamine and sumatriptan [24–26]. Although benefit from sumatriptan for postdural puncture headache has been shown in several case studies and is seen anecdotally in patients with persistent headache despite receiving an epidural blood patch, a small controlled study [$N = 10$] of sumatriptan given to patients scheduled for epidural blood patch failed to confirm benefit [27].

> **Pearl for the practitioner:**
> Do not use treatment response to make a headache diagnosis. Serious, secondary headaches may be temporarily relieved with sumatriptan or other migraine therapies.

Trap 3. Failing to Recognize Secondary Headache

Chapter 3 is devoted to the topic of secondary headaches. Patients known to have a primary headache diagnosis may seek care in the ED due to an exacerbation of their primary headache or for a new, secondary headache. Secondary headaches are easiest to overlook in patients who frequently seek ED care for their established primary headaches.

> ***Pearl for the practitioner:***
> A key question to ask is, "Why did this patient with chronic headaches present to the ED *today?*"

A question typically posed to patients presenting to the ED for headache is: "*Is this your worst headache?*" That question is intended to distinguish if the current headache is significantly different from usual headaches, possibly suggesting an important secondary headache. While this sounds straightforward, studies suggest that patient responses are often inaccurate and fail to correctly identify new or unusual headaches. In an interesting study, ED doctors at the University of New Mexico School of Medicine asked adult patients seen in the ED for a chief complaint of headache five questions, two of which related to headache severity and three of which were distracter questions [28]. The results of this study showed that asking about worst headache often produces inaccurate results (Table 1.3):

- Only 38% of those patients reporting that this was their worst headache not had a bad headache like this in the past, meaning it actually was their "worst headache."
- 62% of patients reporting that this was the worst headache in their lives also gave an example of a similarly severe headache occurring in the past.

In some cases, patients may be saying that this is the worst headache because their previous headaches may have been of this same severity but never worse than the current headache. While attending to complaints of "worst headache" is important so that secondary headaches are not missed, merely hearing that this is the worst headache of the patient's life does not mean that headache is necessarily due to an ominous cause. Additional questions to understand why this headache is considered "worst" are important.

> ***Pearl for the practitioner:***
> Patients reporting having the "worst headache of my life" will need additional follow-up questions to accurately determine how the quality and severity of the current headache relates to previous headache episodes.

Table 1.3 Agreement between questions asked to 60 adult ED headache patients who were queried about headache severity (based on [28])

		When was the last time you had a headache that was this bad?		
		Never	Time given	Total
Is this the worst headache of your life?	Yes	14	23	37
	No	1	22	23
Total		15	45	60

Patients for whom responses to the questions appropriately agreed are shown in the gray boxes. Although both questions are similar, 40% of patients provided responses that failed to show agreement between these two queries about worst headache. This study highlights that reports of "the worst headache of my life" can be unreliable for predicting ominous causes of headache

Trap 4. Failing to Identify Traumatic Headache

While nontraumatic headaches are usually benign, primary headaches, traumatic headaches generally require a more intensive work-up, including imaging studies of the head and neck. In some cases, trauma may be unreported (e.g., from abused children, abused or confused elders, or those with unwitnessed trauma). Suspicious behavior from caregivers or spouses, evidence of current or previous trauma, or an insufficient history may necessitate additional testing to ensure that unreported trauma did not contribute to the current headache complaints.

Trap 5. Failing to Address Hypertension Appropriately

Hypertension is often overlooked in the ED. In one study, only 57% of patients presenting to the ED with a blood pressure >140 mmHg systolic or 90 mmHg diastolic had their blood pressure reassessed during the same visit [29]. Patients were over twice as likely to have a repeat blood pressure when the ED had a blood pressure reassessment protocol. Furthermore, a survey of patients seen in the ED with severe hypertension (systolic blood pressure >180 mmHg or diastolic pressures >110 mmHg) showed that fundoscopic assessment was completed in only 36% of patients, blood work in 73%, an electrocardiogram in 53%, a chest x-ray in 46%, and a urinalysis in 43% [30]. These data show that hypertension is often incompletely assessed in the ED. With the utilization of electronic medical records in the ED, built-in decision support tools can remind clinicians to repeat elevated blood pressures and to perform a fundoscopic exam if blood pressure remains elevated.

Hypertension may occur comorbidly with primary headaches. Migraine sufferers are 40% more likely to have comorbid hypertension compared with headache-free controls [31]. Furthermore, patients with primary headaches occurring more than 15 days per month are twice as likely to have hypertension requiring treatment

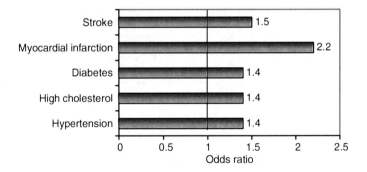

Fig. 1.4 Odds ratios for cardiovascular risk factors and disease in migraineurs vs. controls (based on [31]). Odds >1 represent higher risk among migraineurs. Each variable was significantly increased in migraine sufferers

compared with patients with infrequent primary headaches [32]. Migraineurs are also at a significantly higher risk for cardiovascular disease and other risk factors, so identifying and treating hypertension in this population is particularly important (Fig. 1.4) [31].

> **Pearl for the practitioner:**
> Hypertension should not be routinely attributed to headache pain. Elevated blood pressure should be repeated. Persistently elevated blood pressure will need to be explored directly.

During acute pain episodes, like severe primary headaches, patients may have an elevation in blood pressure. Whether the headache is caused by hypertension or blood pressure elevations are the result of severe head pain can be unclear. In an interesting study, patients with no history of hypertension who had an initial blood pressure at the ED >140 mmHg systolic or 90 mmHg diastolic and an elevated repeated pressure during the same visit were asked to monitor blood pressures at home twice daily for 1 week [33]. Among those patients with elevated blood pressures in the ED, 51% continued to record blood pressure elevations at home. Surprisingly, higher levels of pain or anxiety during the ED visit did not predict lower blood pressures once the patient was home. Therefore, hypertension during an ED headache visit should not be automatically attributed to pain.

The relationship of expected symptoms with elevated blood pressure has also been called into question. In a novel study, records from consecutive patients seen in the ED with hypertension were reviewed for the presence of typical hypertension-related symptoms [34]. Headache occurred in one-third of patients with hypertension, but headache was unrelated to blood pressure severity (Fig. 1.5). The only symptom that did occur significantly more often as blood pressure elevation increased was dyspnea, which was a chief complaint in 8% with stage 1 hypertension, 10% with stage 2, and 20% with stage 3 ($P=0.004$). See Table 1.4 for hypertension definitions [35]. In order to avoid incorrectly attributing elevated blood pressure to hypertension in

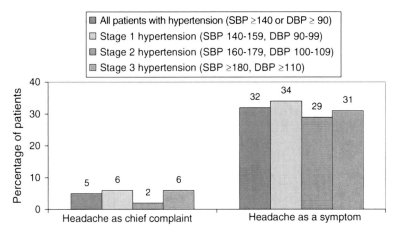

Fig. 1.5 Headache is unrelated to severity of blood pressure elevations (based on [34]). *DBP* diastolic blood pressure, *SBP* systolic blood pressure. Blood pressure values are all mmHg

Table 1.4 Hypertension definitions (based on [35])

Stage	Systolic blood pressure (mmHg)	Diastolic blood pressure (mmHg)
1	140–159	90–99
2	160–179	100–109
3	≥180	≥110

Note: The JNC will release their eighth report in the fall of 2011

patients for whom pain may be the cause of acute elevations, blood pressures should be repeated after pain-relieving treatments have been implemented and monitored throughout the ED visit.

> **Pearl for the practitioner:**
> While the link between acute blood pressure elevations and head pain is unclear, identifying and arranging follow-up for hypertension in ED patients with headache may be especially important in migraine patients who are at significantly higher risk for cardiovascular disease than non-headache controls.

ED Visits for Headache Can Lead to Unnecessary Admissions

Although most nontraumatic headache visits to the ED are for primary headaches that will be discharged from the ED, an important and costly minority of these patients are admitted to the hospital. A large survey identified headache not related to trauma, inflammation, intracranial infection, increased pressure, or mass lesion, or other serious illness in 2% (*N* = 80,500) of ED visits over a 1-year period in

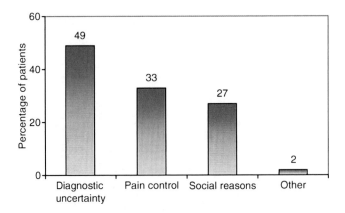

Fig. 1.6 Reasons for admission from ED for headache (based on [36]). Patients could endorse >1 reason

Singapore [36]. Among all of these headache patients, 18% were admitted, most commonly for diagnostic uncertainty and pain control (Fig. 1.6). Patients were admitted for an average of slightly more than 2.5 days, with a range from 1 to 35 days. Discharge diagnoses were most commonly migraine (29%), tension-type headache (25%), nonspecific headache (16%), and cervicogenic headache (8%). A potentially serious diagnosis was given to only 8% of patients, including hemorrhage, stroke, infection, hydrocephalus, seizure, and metastatic disease. These data support that, with better education, evaluation, and treatment protocols, and close follow up by headache-interested providers, many hospital admissions from the ED for headache might be avoided.

> **Pearl for the practitioner:**
> Hospitalization of headache patients from the ED occurs most commonly due to diagnostic uncertainty. Among those patients hospitalized, <10% are eventually diagnosed with significant pathology.

Streamlining the ED for Efficient and Effective Care of Headache Patients

The primary goals of ED headache management are to:

- Determine whether the headache is primary (usually migraine) or secondary. Making the specific diagnosis of which type of primary headache is less important.

  - Rule out important secondary causes of headache
  - Understand unique aspects of headache in children, pregnant and nursing women, and older patients

Box 1.2 Tenets of Headache Care in the ED

1. ED staff should recognize that patient concerns prompting an ED visit for chronic headache may conflict with their own view of what constitutes the need for emergency care.
2. Headache patients should be provided with compassionate care delivered as promptly as possible.
3. A focused history and physical, including a good screening neurological exam, can direct the need for additional testing.
4. The headache assessment should include consideration of rare secondary causes of headache.
5. Distinguishing primary from secondary headache is more important than trying to clarify which specific primary headache diagnosis should be assigned to an individual patient.
6. Selective use of imaging procedures and other testing should be used to rule out rare, secondary causes of headaches.
7. Patients with protracted, primary headaches often need to be rehydrated.
8. Nausea should be treated aggressively.
9. Headache-specific treatments and effective nonopioid analgesics should be used to target headache pain, without an over-reliance on narcotic medications. In general, opioids should not be routinely used as part of an interim treatment strategy after ED discharge as other effective, less problematic options are available.
10. Clear, written, take-home instructions should be given to patients to describe: how to manage continuing or recurring headaches; how to contact a primary care provider or other headache-interested provider for ongoing care; and when to return to the ED.
11. Patient instruction sheets on general headache treatment and prevention tips should be provided to help facilitate effective self-management of chronic headaches to minimize reliance on the ED for headache symptoms.
12. Follow-up should be arranged with a primary care provider or headache-interested doctor within 1–2 weeks of ED discharge.

- Provide sufficient analgesia to reduce headache symptoms to a more tolerable level.
- Treat nausea aggressively.
- Develop an effective interim treatment plan with appropriate medications to last until the patient can see his/her outpatient healthcare provider.
- Facilitate post-ED follow-up care for ongoing headache complaints.
- Prevent unnecessary repeat ED visits for headache patients.

Consistently utilizing a streamlined approach to headache patient assessment and treatment can maximize effective treatment, improve staff and patient satisfaction, and minimize ED recidivism (Box 1.2).

Subsequent chapters will address these goals in greater detail and provide practical recommendations for the care of ED headache patients. Sample discharge instructions, including general information on primary headache management and headaches after minor head injury, are provided. Specific chapters will deal with special populations of patients including children and adolescents, pregnant and lactating women, and the older adult with headaches. By using simple and practical assessment and treatment tools, including questionnaires and clinical algorithms, headache patients can be efficiently and effectively treated in a busy ED. The practical tools contained in the book may be photocopied from the pages of this book or downloaded from http://extras.springer.com/. You may also be linked directly to these downloads through a link at http://www.dawnmarcusmd.com.

Summary

- Nearly two of every three patients evaluated in emergency settings for nontraumatic headache will be diagnosed with a benign or primary headache disorder, usually migraine.
- A specific primary headache diagnosis will not be able to be determined for one in four patients with a primary headache seen in the ED.
- Secondary headaches in the ED are more common in middle and older aged adults, especially those >75 years of age.
- ED care of migraine is expensive, costing nearly $2,000 per patient visit. Many of these visits – especially repeat visits – can be avoided with a good interim treatment strategy and outpatient headache care.
- Assessment errors commonly encountered in the ED management of headache include:
  - Spending too much time to determine which type of primary headache should be assigned
  - Using treatment response to determine a headache diagnosis
  - Not understanding the meaning of reports of the "worst headache of my life"
  - Failure to identify unreported trauma
  - Failure to appropriately address hypertension
- Nearly half of all hospital admissions for headache from the ED are caused by diagnostic uncertainty. A well thought out approach to evaluation of the patient with an acute headache can reduce admissions related to diagnostic uncertainty.
- Only 8% of patients hospitalized for headache from the ED are eventually diagnosed with significant pathology.
- Patients – but not ED staff – often consider having symptoms outside of business hours to constitute an indication for ED care.
- Improving access to and utilization of outpatient primary care or other headache-interested providers may substantially reduce unnecessary repeat ED visits for acute headache treatment.

References

1. McCaig LF, Nawar EW. National Hospital Ambulatory Medical Care Survey. 2004 emergency department summary. Adv Data. 2006;372:1–29.
2. http://www.neurologyreviews.com/sep06/headache.html. Accessed Jun 2010.
3. American Board of Emergency Medicine website. http://www.abem.org. Accessed Jun 2010.
4. Headache Classification Subcommittee of the International Headache Society. The international classification of headache disorders. 2nd edition. Cephalalgia. 2004;24 Suppl 1:1–160.
5. Fiesseler FW, Riggs RL, Holubek W, Eskin B, Richman PB. Canadian Headache Society criteria for the diagnosis of acute migraine headache in the ED – do our patients meet these criteria? Am J Emerg Med. 2005;23:149–54.
6. Goldstein JN, Camargo CA, Pelletier AJ, Edlow JA. Headache in the United States emergency departments: demographics, work-up and frequency of pathological disease. Cephalalgia. 2006;26:684–90.
7. Friedman BW, Serrano D, Reed M, Diamond M, Lipton RB. Use of the emergency department for severe headache. A population-based study. Headache. 2009;49:21–30.
8. Friedman D, Feldon S, Holloway R, Fisher S. Utilization, diagnosis, treatment and cost of migraine treatment in the emergency department. Headache. 2009;49:1163–73.
9. Gupta MX, Silberstein SD, Young WB, et al. Less is not more: underutilization of headache medications in a university hospital emergency department. Headache. 2007;47:1125–33.
10. Cydulka RK, Korte R. Career satisfaction in emergency medicine: the ABEM Longitudinal Study of Emergency Physicians. Ann Emerg Med. 2008;51:714–22.
11. Kuhn G, Goldberg R, Compton S. Tolerance of uncertainty, burnout, and satisfaction with the career of emergency medicine. Ann Emerg Med. 2009;54:106–13.
12. Derlet RW, Ledesma A. How do prudent laypeople define an emergency medical condition? J Emerg Med. 1999;17:413–8.
13. Swadron SP. Pitfalls in the management of headache in the emergency department. Emerg Med Clin N Am. 2010;28:127–47.
14. Vargas BB. Tension-type headache and migraine: two points on a continuum? Curr Pain Headache Rep. 2008;12:433–6.
15. Friedman BW, Hochberg ML, Esses D, et al. Applying the International Classification of Headache Disorders to the emergency department: an assessment of reproducibility and the frequency with which a unique diagnosis can be assigned to every acute headache presentation. Ann Emerg Med. 2007;49:409–19.
16. Miner JR, Smith SW, Moore J, Biros M. Sumatriptan for the treatment of undifferentiated primary headaches in the ED. Am J Emerg Med. 2007;25:60–4.
17. Trainor A, Miner J. Pain treatment and relief among patients with primary headache subtypes in the ED. Am J Emerg Med. 2008;26:1029–34.
18. Law S, Derry S, Moore RA. Triptans for acute cluster headache. Cochrane Database Syst Rev. 2010;4:CD008042.
19. Prokhorov S, Khanna S, Alapati D, Pallimalli SL. Subcutaneous sumatriptan relieved migraine-like headache in two adolescents with aseptic meningitis. Headache. 2008;48:1235–6.
20. Pfadenhauer K, Schönsteiner T, Keller H. The risks of sumatriptan administration in patients with unrecognized subarachnoid haemorrhage (SAH). Cephalalgia. 2006;26:320–33.
21. Evans RW, Davenport RJ. Benign or sinister? Distinguishing migraine from subarachnoid hemorrhage. Headache. 2007;47:433–5.
22. Leira EC, Cruz-Flores S, Leacock RO, Abdulrauf SI. Sumatriptan can alleviate headaches due to carotid artery dissection. Headache. 2001;41:590–1.
23. Manfredi PL, Shenoy S, Payne R. Sumatriptan for headache caused by head and neck cancer. Headache. 2000;40:758–60.
24. Hodgson C, Roitberg-Henry A. The use of sumatriptan in the treatment of postdural puncture headache. Anaesthesia. 1997;52:808.

25. Ward TN, Levin M. Case reports: headache caused by a spinal cord stimulator in the upper cervical spine. Headache. 2000;40:689–91.
26. Koul R, Chacko A, Javed H, et al. Syndrome of cerebrospinal fluid hypovolemia following lumbar puncture cerebrospinal fluid leak in a patient with idiopathic intracranial hypertension. J Child Neurol. 2002;17:77–9.
27. Connelly NR, Parker RK, Rahimi A, Gibson CS. Sumatriptan in patients with postdural puncture headache. Headache. 2000;40:316–9.
28. Diaz M, Braude D, Skipper B. Concordance of historical questions used in risk-stratifying patients with headache. Am J Emerg Med. 2007;25:907–10.
29. Baumann BM, Cline DM, Cienki JJ, et al. Provider self-report and practice: reassessment and referral of emergency department patients with elevated blood pressures. Am J Hypertens. 2009;22:604–10.
30. Karras DJ, Kruus LK, Cienki JJ, et al. Evaluation and treatment of patients with severely elevated blood pressure in academic emergency departments: a multicenter study. Ann Emerg Med. 2006;47:230–6.
31. Bigal ME, Kurth T, Santanello N, et al. Migraine and cardiovascular disease: a population-based study. Neurology. 2010;74:628–35.
32. Gipponi S, Venturelli E, Rao R, Liberini P, Padovani A. Hypertension is a factor associated with chronic daily headache. Neurol Sci. 2010;31 Suppl 1:S171–3.
33. Tanabe P, Persell SD, Adams JG, et al. Increased blood pressure in the emergency department: pain, anxiety, or undiagnosed hypertension? Ann Emerg Med. 2008;51:221–9.
34. Karras DJ, Ufberg JW, Harrigan RA, et al. Lack of relationship between hypertension-associated symptoms and blood pressure in hypertensive ED patients. Am J Emerg Med. 2005;23:106–10.
35. 7th report of the joint national committee on prevention, detection, evaluation, and treatment of high blood pressure. Available at the National Heart, Lung, and Blood Institute website http://www.nhlbi.nih.gov. Accessed Jan 2011.
36. Ang SH, Chan YC, Mah M. Emergency department headache admission in an acute care hospital: why do they occur and what can we do about it? Ann Acad Med Sing. 2009;38:1007–10.

Chapter 2
Getting Started

Key Chapter Points

- Headaches caused by readily identifiable, underlying conditions (e.g., trauma, meningitis, subarachnoid hemorrhage, etc.) are called secondary headaches. Primary headaches are headaches without a readily identifiable, underlying medical condition (e.g., migraine, tension-type, and cluster headaches).
- ED headache diagnosis should focus on differentiating primary from secondary headache, rather than determining a specific primary headache diagnosis.
- Six essential questions can help determine why patients are presenting to the ED and whether they are likely to have a secondary headache.
- An effective, focused screening neurological examination can generally be performed in about 5 minutes.
- Imaging studies are usually unnecessary for patients with chronic headaches without alarm signs or symptoms.
- Patients >50 years old with a new headache should be screened for giant cell arteritis. Other causes, such as primary and metastatic cancers may also need to be considered.

Keywords Computed tomography • Lumbar puncture • Magnetic resonance imaging • Spinal fluid

---

Box 2.1 Case

Janet is a 32-year-old legal secretary who came to the ED after work with a "splitting headache." During her visit, "The doctor asked me so many questions, I just started saying 'yes' to everything so he'd finish and they could give me my usual migraine medicine. My regular doctor told me that if I get a bad headache after office hours that doesn't get better with my usual pills,

---

(continued)

D.A. Marcus and P.A. Bain, *Practical Assessment and Treatment of the Patient*   21
with Headaches in the Emergency Department and Urgent Care Clinic,
DOI 10.1007/978-1-4614-0002-8_2, © Springer Science+Business Media, LLC 2011

Box 2.1 (continued)

to just come to the emergency room so they can treat it before it really gets out of hand and I'm stuck in bed for days! I assumed they knew I've done this a couple of times a year." After 6 hours, a brain scan, spinal tap, blood cultures, and other blood work, Janet is frustrated and angry. "I've been here for hours already and I still haven't gotten any treatment!"

Box 2.2 Main Tasks for ED Personnel Treating Patients with Headache

1. Rule out secondary headaches
2. Provide symptomatic relief
3. Make sure the patient has appropriate follow-up

The emergency department (ED) staff is often tasked with the difficult job of determining whether ED headaches are patient's typical, severe chronic headache or a new, possibly secondary headache signifying important underlying pathology that might need urgent treatment. Patients typically avoid ED visits for chronic headache until severe and usual treatments have failed; at that point, patients like Janet may also become reluctant historians, more interested in getting symptomatic relief than providing accurate and complete historical information to the ED staff.

Every patient presenting to the ED for headache will need to be assessed with a focused history and physical examination. The primary objective of the ED headache evaluation is to differentiate primary (e.g., migraine, tension-type, or cluster headache) from secondary (e.g., headaches due to specific medical conditions, such as meningitis, subarachnoid hemorrhage [SAH], or giant cell [temporal] arteritis) headaches. Patients with a primary headache may be treated symptomatically, with outpatient follow-up arranged following ED discharge. Patients with possible secondary headaches will require a more extensive work-up in the ED. Secondary headaches will be reviewed in detail in Chap. 3.

Why Focus on Primary vs. Secondary Headaches?

The ED staff needs to ensure that patients requiring urgent treatment for secondary headaches get the workup and care they need. In some cases, the workup may need to be completed after discharge from the ED. In most cases, the ED staff can effectively determine which patients have secondary headaches. The ED, however, is not an ideal environment for distinguishing among various types of primary headache. In one study, ED reviewers agreed on whether ED patients with nontraumatic headache should be diagnosed with a secondary headache in 94% of cases and a primary headache in 91% of cases [1]. Although there was excellent agreement about differentiating primary from secondary headache, 26% of those patients identified as having some type of primary headache could not be given a specific headache diagnosis. Assigning a specific primary headache diagnosis requires a detailed review of the patient's typical headache pattern, which may be different from the headache that brought the patient to the ED. In many cases, a correct diagnosis cannot be arrived at until several weeks worth of headache diary recordings have been reviewed and several patient interviews have been conducted. Patients in acute distress are often poor and incomplete historians, so an ED-assigned diagnosis may need to be revised when a patient is able to provide more complete information during outpatient follow-up assessment.

> ***Pearl for the practitioner:***
> ED headache assessment should focus on differentiating primary from secondary headache rather than identifying a specific primary headache diagnosis.

Important Questions to Ask in the ED

Patient responses to six essential ED headache questions (Box 2.3) help categorize them into one of four major headache categories (Figs. 2.1 and 2.2):

1. Patients with a new headache
2. Patients with a chronic headache
3. Patients with a headache PLUS other symptoms or signs
4. Headache in patients with known and likely contributory medical illnesses

> **Box 2.3** Six Essential Questions to Ask Patients Being Seen in the ED for Headaches
>
> 1. Have you had any head injury within the last week?
> 2. What specifically happened that made you come to the ED for your headache today?
> 3. Have you had similar headaches before?
> 4. How long did it take for today's headache to reach its greatest intensity? (Record in seconds, minutes, or hours.)
> 5. Is anything else bothering you besides the headache?
> 6. Do you have any other medical problems, such as cancer, human immunodeficiency virus (HIV), or other serious medical illnesses?

Fig. 2.1 Defining headache
category based on six
essential questions

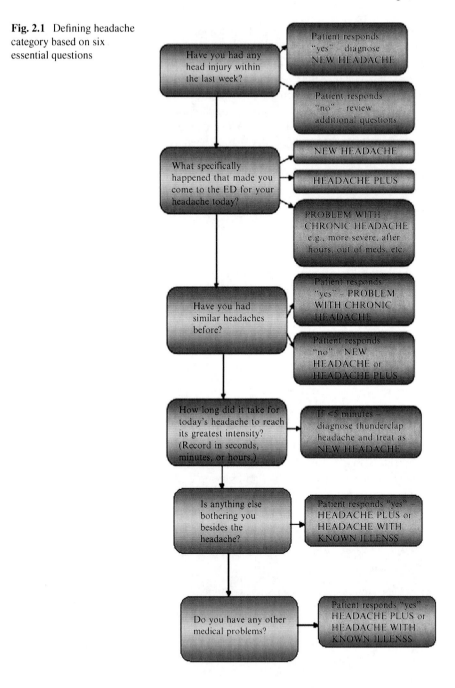

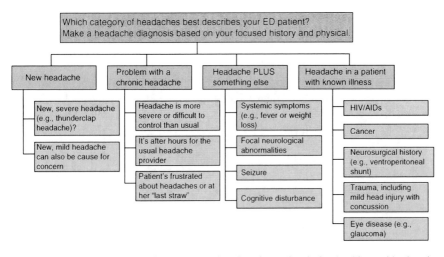

Fig. 2.2 Diagnostic algorithm for probable chronic primary headache (problem with chronic headache) vs. secondary headaches (new headache, headache plus, or headache with illness) in the ED. *AIDS* acquired immune deficiency syndrome, *HIV* human immunodeficiency virus

Information may be gathered on a standardized form (Box 2.4)

Headaches beginning suddenly AND reaching peak intensity within seconds to minutes are called *thunderclap headache*. In one study, 100% of patients presenting to the ED with sudden onset, severe headache who were eventually diagnosed with a SAH had their headache reach its peak within 5 min [2]. Quantifying *time-to-peak severity* rather than more vague descriptors is important when trying to identify if patients have potentially worrisome thunderclap headache. Reports of "headache started suddenly" do not necessarily equate with "instantly severe [2]."

> **Pearl for the practitioner:**
> Sudden onset, severe headaches reaching peak intensity in ≤5 min are *thunderclap headaches*. These headaches need careful evaluation to rule our subarachnoid hemorrhage, usually requiring noncontrast brain computed tomography (CT) *AND* spinal tap to rule out blood in the cerebrospinal fluid (CSF) or xanthochromia (yellowish discoloration of the CSF due to blood breakdown products).

Those patients with (1) a new headache (which will include most cases of thunderclap headache), (2) headache PLUS, or (3) headache with known illness will need a more extensive evaluation for possible secondary headaches. This checklist of six questions can be asked by nonphysician ED personnel and confirmed by physicians for increased efficiency.

Box 2.4 Headache History Collection Form

Patient name:_____
Date: _____

1. Have you had any head injury within the last week? YES NO
2. What specifically happened that made you come to the ED for your headache today?

   _____
   _____

3. Have you had similar headaches before? YES NO
4. How long did it take for today's headache to reach its greatest intensity?
   (record in seconds, minutes, or hours) _____
5. Is anything else bothering you besides the headache? Have you recently
   had seizures, vomiting, fever, weight loss, or other problems?

   _____
   _____

6. Do you have any other medical problems, such as cancer, HIV, or other
   serious medical illnesses?

   _____
   _____

Additional history:

1. Are you or could you be pregnant? YES NO Record method of contraception _____
2. Are you breastfeeding? YES NO
3. What medications do you take?

   _____
   _____

4. What medications (including over-the-counter, prescription, and any street
   drugs) have you used in the last 24 h?

   _____
   _____

5. Do you have any allergies?

   _____
   _____

Patients with a New Headache

New headache may occur with secondary headaches as well as the initial presentation of a new, primary headache. Additional evaluation is usually needed in patients with a new headache before a diagnosis of primary headache can be given.

While severe headaches that begin suddenly, the so-called thunderclap headache, raise concern about SAH, many other causes of thunderclap headache have been identified (Box 2.5 and Fig. 2.3) [3]. Any new headache – mild or severe, gradual onset or abrupt – can, however, be cause for concern and will need a more extensive evaluation.

Box 2.5 Secondary Headaches Causing Sudden, Severe, or Thunderclap-Type Headache

- Acute hypertensive crisis
- Vascular disease

  - Hemorrhage, e.g., extradural, intradural, subarachnoid, or intracranial hemorrhage
  - Thrombosis, e.g., cerebral venous sinus thrombosis
  - Carotid or vertebral artery dissection
  - Cerebrovascular accident
  - Pituitary apoplexy

- Infection

  - Systemic infection
  - Meningitis
  - Encephalitis

- Intracranial mass

  - Third ventricle tumor obstructing CSF drainage, e.g., colloid cyst

- Low intracranial pressure

  - Spontaneous intracranial hypotension
  - Dural tear at spinal nerve root

Patients with a Chronic Headache

Remember – patients may have a chronic, primary headache AND also a new, secondary headache. Before diagnosing a patients with a chronic, primary headache, make sure you understand WHY they came to the ED for this particular headache. If there are new features to a chronic headache (e.g., new development of a migraine aura), additional evaluation may be needed to rule out a coexisting secondary headache.

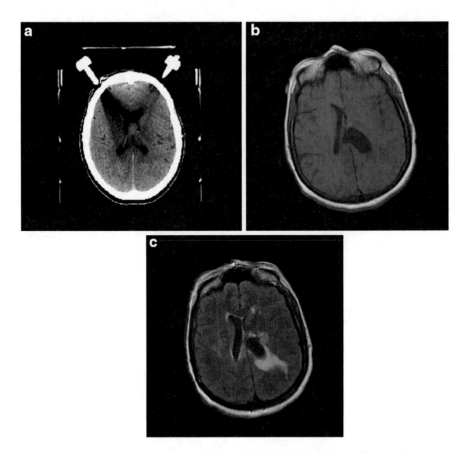

Fig. 2.3 Colloid cyst (images courtesy of Clayton A. Wiley, MD, PhD). (**a**) Computed tomography scan, horizontal view. This intra-operative scan of a patient with a third ventricular colloid cyst shows the patient's head immobilized within a stereotactic frame, with two pins visible at 11 and 1 o'clock that cast shadows in the brain image. In the center of the brain, sandwiched between the dark cerebral ventricles, is a gray oval mass. This mass proved to be a benign colloid cyst whose size eventually blocked the outflow of cerebrospinal fluid from the ventricles. Once the size had enlarged sufficiently to block flow from the ventricles, the patient developed severe headaches. (**b**) Magnetic resonance, T-1 weighted horizontal image after surgery. Postoperative imaging after removal of the colloid cyst shows swelling of the brain on the right side of the figure with asymmetric compression of the lateral ventricle. (**c**) Magnetic resonance, T-2 weighted horizontal image after surgery. Using a different signal sequence, excess fluid can be noted on the right side of the figure in the brain tissue surrounding the lateral ventricles. This bright signal is consistent with brain edema and swelling

Pearl for the practitioner:

An important pitfall in history taking is assuming that patients with a chronic headache – e.g., migraine – will only present to the ED with that diagnosis. Always consider other causes of headaches, even when patients have an established history of migraine. Asking what brought the patient to the ED TODAY can be helpful in sorting out whether or not a new headache type is present.

Patients with Self-Reported "Sinus Headache"

Autonomic features (e.g., lacrimation and rhinorrhea) are frequently reported by patients with migraine. Frequent occurrence of mild autonomic features in many migraineurs may result in incorrectly attributing migraines to cluster headache or, more commonly, sinus disease. Evaluation of 100 consecutive patients with self-diagnosed "sinus" headache determined that 85% had migraine, while only 3% actually had headache associated with rhinosinusitis [4]. Among patients with definite migraine, several headache features were reported that resulted in the false attribution of headache to the sinuses (Fig. 2.4). Furthermore, migraine headaches will often respond to treatment with antihistamines, perpetuating the frequent false perception that the headaches are caused by sinus pathology. Autonomic features in migraine may also occur consistently with attacks and affect only one side of the face, adding to the confusion with cluster or sinus headaches. A large community survey ($N = 841$) reported at least one *unilateral* autonomic symptom *regularly* occurred during typical

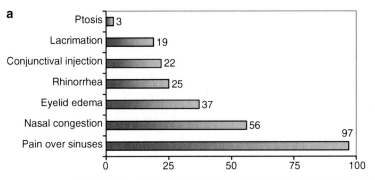

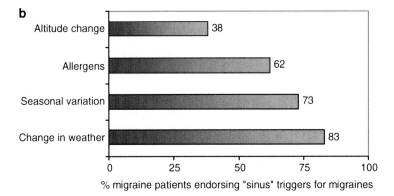

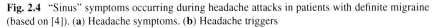

Fig. 2.4 "Sinus" symptoms occurring during headache attacks in patients with definite migraine (based on [4]). (**a**) Headache symptoms. (**b**) Headache triggers

migraine attacks for one in four migraineurs [5]. In another large study ($N = 2,991$), 88% of patients with self-reported or physician-diagnosed "sinus" headache were found to actually have migraine as the cause of their headache pain [6].

A good rule of thumb is that when a patient presents with a fever, discolored and/ or bloody nasal discharge, and has a headache as a secondary feature, the headache may well be related to acute sinusitis. When headache is the predominant symptom, it is far more likely to be a migraine headache than acute sinusitis.

> *Pearl for the practitioner:*
> Due to the frequent occurrence of mild autonomic symptoms and pain located over the sinuses with migraine, patients often incorrectly label their migraines as "sinus" headaches.

Now That I've Diagnosed a Primary Headache, How Do I Know If It's Migraine?

Most patients with a primary headache in the ED will have migraine. Once secondary causes of headache are ruled out, ED patients with a primary headache diagnosis can complete the three item, validated ID-Migraine screener [7]. This screening tool can help to confirm patients with a likely diagnosis of migraine and patients should be encouraged to share the results with their primary provider (Box 2.6). In one study, sensitivity and specificity for accurately diagnosing migraine were 0.94 and 0.83, respectively, among ED patients identified with primary headache [8]. Unfortunately, 29% of patients with secondary headaches were incorrectly identified as having migraine using this screener and all patients with cluster headache were incorrectly classified as having migraine. Therefore, the ID-Migraine screener should only be given to patients already determined to have a primary headache. Furthermore, patients should understand that the diagnosis given from this screening tool is only a preliminary assessment and a more detailed evaluation with their outpatient provider will be needed to confirm the diagnosis of migraine. The authors from this study recommended using the screener as a final check after the full ED evaluation had been completed to facilitate identification of migraine and incorrectly limit assigning a "nonspecific headache" diagnosis to patients with migraine.

> *Pearl for the practitioner:*
> Once secondary headaches have been ruled out, the three-item ID-Migraine screener can effectively and efficiently confirm that migraine is the likely diagnosis.

Box 2.6 ID-Migraine Screener (Adapted from [7])

Answer the following three questions about your headaches:

1. Over the last 3 months, have you limited your activities on at least 1 day because of your headaches?
2. Do lights bother you when you have a headache?
3. Do you get sick to your stomach or nauseated with your headache?

If you answered "yes" to at least two of these questions, you probably have migraine.

Cutaneous allodynia is frequently assessed headache clinics. Cutaneous allodynia describes a hypersensitivity to touch stimulation so that normally nonpainful touch stimuli invoke a pain response. A good example of cutaneous allodynia is a sunburn. Before experiencing the burn, touching the skin does not produce pain. Once a sunburn has occurred, normally nonpainful touch produces pain. Migraineurs frequently describe cutaneous allodynia, reporting pain with brushing the hair or when wearing hats, glasses, earrings, or tight clothing during a migraine. Cutaneous allodynia is endorsed by at least 60% of migraineurs attending headache clinics [9, 10] and is often recommended to be included as part of the routine outpatient migraine evaluation [11, 12]. Cutaneous allodynia, however, is infrequently seen in migraine patients presenting to the ED, with only 14% having allodynia in one ED study [13]. Therefore, allodynia assessment is not recommended for ED primary headache. Early work by Dr. Rami Burstein resulted in the promotion of early migraine treatment before allodynia had occurred, called "the race to allodynia." Burstein's work showed that migraine treatment with sumatriptan was most successful when the drug had been administered prior to the development of cutaneous allodynia [14, 15]. More recent studies, however, have disputed the need to treat prior to the onset of allodynia with two other triptans (almotriptan and rizatriptan) [16–18] and dihydroergotamine (DHE) [19, 20].

Patients with a Headache PLUS Other Symptoms or Signs

Patients presenting with evidence of systemic or neurological illness (e.g., fever, weight loss, paresis, or seizures) will require additional testing. These patients are probably least likely to leave the ED with a diagnosis of a primary headache and will require the most complete assessment during their ED visit as well as closer outpatient follow-up with their primary care or other headache-interested provider.

Headache in Patients with Known and Likely Contributory Medical Illnesses

Headache is a common symptom occurring in a wide range of medical problems. Evaluation of patients with known or likely-to-be contributing medical illnesses will need evaluations targeted to those specific identified illnesses. Patients with headaches who have a known history of malignancy or human immunodeficiency virus (HIV) should have evaluations for brain metastases or infections that occur with higher frequency in immune compromised patients. Patients with headache beginning after trauma should be diagnosed with post-traumatic headache and will need additional testing to determine the severity of their traumatic injuries.

Box 2.7 Concussion Assessment Questions

1. Did you get knocked out?
2. Did you feel dazed, see stars, or "get the wind knocked out of you?"
3. Did observers see the patient get knocked out or seem confused or dazed after the head injury?
4. Do you remember the injury occurring and events right before and after the injury?

If the patient or those who observed the injury can answer "yes" to any of the first three questions OR "no" to the fourth question, diagnose a concussion.

Traumatic Headache

Concussion is generally defined as any alteration of mental function following a blow to the head that may or may not involve a frank loss of consciousness. Patients who report *any* head injury should be screened for evidence of a concussion (Box 2.7). Patients reporting headache after trauma also require additional testing to determine the extent of their injuries. The Glasgow coma scale (GCS) is a routine measure of acute brain injury severity, with possible scores from 3 to 15 (Table 2.1). The GSC and other features are used to determine whether the head injury should be considered to be mild or not (Box 2.8).

About 7–8% of patients having a mild head injury have been shown to have abnormalities on computed tomography (CT) imaging [21, 22]. Factors associated with abnormal CT imaging after mild head injury are listed in Table 2.2. GCS is strongly linked to imaging abnormalities; abnormal CT scans occur in about 5% of patients with GCS of 15% vs. 30% when the GCS is 13 [23]. Patients with none of

Table 2.1 Glasgow coma scale

Category	Action	Score
Eye opening	Spontaneous	4
	To speech	3
	To pain	2
	None	1
Best motor reaction	Obeys verbal commands	6
	Localizes pain	5
	Flexion to pain – withdrawal	4
	Flexion to pain – abnormal	3
	Extension to pain	2
	None	1
Best verbal reaction	Oriented, converses	5
	Disoriented, converses	4
	Inappropriate words	3
	Incomprehensible words	2
	None	1

Total score (add 3 scores for total)

Brain injury severity is classified by total score as:
- Minor ≥13
- Moderate 9–12
- Severe ≤8

Box 2.8 Mild Head Injury Can Be Diagnosed When At Least One of the Following is Present

- The patient felt dazed, disoriented, or confused at the time of the trauma
- The patient lost consciousness for ≤30 min and their Glasgow coma scale score after 30 min is 13–15
- Memory is lost only for events immediately before or within 24 h after the trauma
- If a focal neurological deficit occurred, it resolved within hours

the factors in Table 2.2 or a normal CT with GCS of 15 can usually be discharged with home observation; while patients with an abnormal CT or GCS <15 will generally need to be admitted for observation [23].

The Centers for Disease Control and Prevention website provides updated information on traumatic brain injury, as well as downloadable resources for mild traumatic brain injury screening instruments, a pocket card for quick reference for clinicians, and helpful patient handouts for post-ED care. The website may be accessed at http://www.cdc.gov/traumaticbraininjury/.

Table 2.2 Factors associated with imaging abnormalities after mild head injury (based on [21, 22])

Category	Characteristic
Demographics	Age >60 years
Concussion clues	Loss of consciousness
	Post-trauma amnesia
	Post-trauma seizure
Symptoms	Headache
	Vomiting
Signs	Extracranial lesions
	Focal neurological deficit
	GCS <15
	Skull fracture
Concomitant conditions	Coagulopathy
	Hydrocephalus with shunt insertion

5-min Screening Neuro Exam

A comprehensive, detailed neurological examination can be very helpful to identify specific areas of abnormality within the brain and nervous system. A comprehensive neuro exam is really designed to answer the question, "Where is the lesion?" The ED assessment, however, should focus on determining if pathology is likely rather than focusing on determining the exact lesion location. Consequently, a brief neuro screening examination can be used to help differentiate primary from secondary headaches in the ED headache patient (Table 2.3 and Fig. 2.5).

In patients with nontraumatic headache, a detailed musculoskeletal assessment of the head and neck is not necessary in the ED. In a recently published study, patients with acute headache for whom SAH and meningitis were ruled out were evaluated with a musculoskeletal examination [24]. Assessments of pericranial muscle tenderness and neck mobility were not found to be helpful for distinguishing primary from secondary headaches.

Abnormal vital signs often signify systemic illness; however, hypertension frequently accompanies primary headache, especially in patients with more frequent headaches. Hypertension has also been linked to a transition of headaches from episodic to frequent or daily headaches [25]. In one study, hypertension occurred in 16% of patients with daily headache vs. 7% with episodic migraine ($P < 0.01$) [26]. Furthermore, an elevation in blood pressure frequently accompanies severe pain, anxiety, or headache [27]. Patients with migraine and moderately elevated blood pressure should have their blood pressure rechecked following successful migraine treatment before antihypertensive therapy is instituted [27]. Tachycardia also frequently accompanies severe headache episodes. Fever, if present, should prompt consideration of infections, connective tissue disorders, and/or malignancies.

Table 2.3 The 5-min neuro exam

Feature evaluated	How to check	What to look for and questions to ask
General health assessment	General appraisal of overall appearance	Does the patient look acutely ill?
	Vital signs	Abnormal vital signs (e.g., elevated temperature, hypotension, tachycardia) often suggest systemic illness
General neuro assessment	Observe the patient walking, if they are able to do so. Also observe sitting/lying posture in patients who are unable to get out of bed	For patients who are able to walk: does the patient move symmetrically, with similar movements of the arms and legs on both sides of the body? Does the patient walk with her feet close together, turn easily, and walk in a straight line OR do you see signs of imbalance?
		For patients observed when sitting: do they easily sit upright or do they tend to lean or fall to one side? Do they hold their arms and legs in a similar posture and move them symmetrically while sitting?
Cognitive assessment	This should be performed as part of the history	Was the patient able to complete paperwork during their intake, showing an ability to read, write, and manipulate a pen? Can the patient speak fluently with good use of language? Can the patient tell a coherent story? Does the patient answer your questions well OR is she confused, disoriented, lethargic, or easily distracted?
Eye grounds/ fundoscopic evaluation	Fundoscopic examination	Look for papilledema to suggest increased intracranial pressure. Vascular constriction or nicking or the presence of hemorrhages or yellowish exudates suggests hypertension.
		Venous pulsations, when present, are a sign of normal intracranial pressure; venous pulsations may be absent when pressure is normal or abnormal
Cranial nerve assessment	Cranial nerve testing can be mainly performed during history taking.	Watch the patient's eye and facial movements for symmetry while the patient is talking to you.
	Check visual fields by asking the patient to look at your nose while you wiggle fingers held with your arms held out at the side and placed about equal distance between you and the patient	Assuming you don't have a problem with your visual fields, both you and the patients should be similarly able to see fingers wiggling on both sides during visual field testing

(continued)

Table 2.3 (continued)

Feature evaluated	How to check	What to look for and questions to ask
Extremity testing for strength and sensation	Observe the patient's resting posture and casual movements during history taking. Test muscles in both the proximal and distal arm and leg on both sides for strength. Tap reflexes at the elbows and knees. Stroke the bottom of the foot for a Babinski response. Lightly stroke both sides with your fingers and an open safety pin to test sensation.	Patients who equally position and move both arms and legs will usually have a normal motor screening examination. If you see differences during casual observation, spend more time carefully testing strength and reflexes. Look for evidence of symmetrical responses to both motor and sensory testing. An up going toe on Babinski testing may suggest an upper motor neuron (e.g., brain or spinal cord) lesion and the need for additional testing. Watch patients as they reach for and manipulate items in their environment to notice fine motor skills and coordination

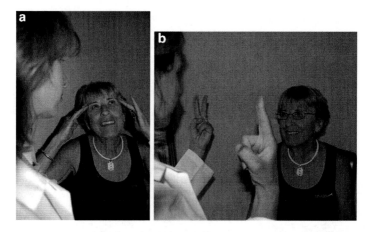

Fig. 2.5 5-min neuro exam. (**a**) Observe patient posture and notice asymmetry in movements of the eyes, face, or extremities while recording the patient's history. (**b**) Place fingers equidistant between examiner and patient for visual field testing. Alternatively, a more detailed visual field examination may be performed by individually testing the ability of patients to identify a stimulus presented to each of four quadrants for each eye. Accurately assessing visual fields in each quadrant can be tedious and is generally unnecessary on a screening exam unless patient complaints suggest a visual abnormality. (**c**) Anchor the ophthalmoscope on the cheek bone for best viewing of the fundus. Once the scope is angled about 45° toward the front of the eye, ask the patient to look forward. When the examiner now looks into the scope, the fundus should be in view or near view. This approach is often more successful than placing the ophthalmoscope first at the examiner's eye and then approaching the patient's eye while viewing through the ophthalmoscope. (**d**) Test strength proximally and distally in all extremities. (**e**) Scrape from the heel on the lateral aspect of the sole toward toes with a dull object. It is generally unnecessary and uncomfortable for the patient to make a full, curving path from the heel, up the side of the foot, and across the top of the sole to the great toe. An up going great toe on Babinski testing suggests brain or spinal cord pathology

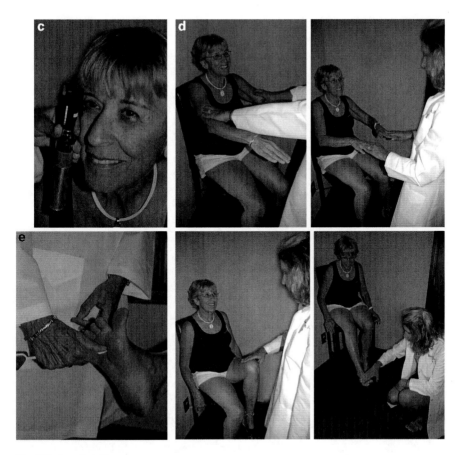

Fig. 2.5 (continued)

Much of the information needed to determine if a patient's nervous system is intact can be gathered by observing the patient during the history-taking portion of the ED assessment. Prior to the formal history taking, the triage nurse and other intake staff have already gathered important information on patient cognition. Additional information is collected by the treating ED staff member by observing how patients respond to questions, maintain a symmetrical posture, and casually move their extremities. The patient should be continuously and carefully observed and assessed throughout all contact time, noting their behavior, eye/facial/and extremity movements, and responses to stimulation. Observation should take precedence over documentation when assessing the headache patient. Even when writing notes, make an effort to attend to the patient and observe him. By focusing on the patient rather than on paperwork, monitors, or other equipment, most of the neuro exam can actually be completed without formally "examining" the patient. For most neurologists, specific cranial nerve, motor, sensory, and balance tests are performed simply to confirm impressions that were already formed through attentive casual observation and to give the patient an impression of being "examined."

> **Pearl for the practitioner:**
> Becoming an active and astute observer during history taking helps the examiner gather important information on neurological functioning that reduces the time needed for formal neurological testing.

It is important to develop a specific sequence for the various steps in the focused neurological exam and do it the same way every time. It may be helpful to write down the sequence in a checklist type format and periodically review it to make sure that all of the important steps are consistently done.

The fundoscopic examination is an important but often neglected part of the neurological screen. In one study of patients reporting to the ED with sudden onset, severe headache, the fundoscopic examination was performed in only 48% of patients [2]. Although magnetic resonance imaging (MRI) and CT scans identify many serious causes of secondary headache, they do not identify all causes of increased intracranial pressure. For example, patients with increased intracranial pressure due to idiopathic intracranial hypertension, previously called pseudotumor cerebri, often have a normal imaging study despite high intracranial pressure. These patients, however, generally have obvious and marked papilledema. Failure to identify these patients can result in significant visual loss. Success with visualizing the fundus is improved by asking the patient to stare forward and anchoring the ophthalmoscope at the patient's cheekbone (Fig. 2.5). Look through the ophthalmoscope keeping both eyes open. The clinician's right eye should look into the patient's right eye. This positioning generally results in good placement to visualize the optic disc. Dimming the light exiting the ophthalmoscope is generally more helpful for minimizing unwanted pupillary constriction compared with reducing room lighting. The fundoscopic examination may be enhanced by using the Welch Allyn Panoptic fundoscope, which provides five times magnification and a 30° wider field of view for easier viewing (details available at http://www.welchallyn.com/promotions/PanOptic). Normal intracranial pressure is supported when vessels exiting the disc are noted to have pulsations (termed *venous pulsations*). The absence of venous pulsations however does not necessarily mean intracranial pressure is increased as venous pulsations may not always be detected in patients with normal intracranial pressure.

Deciding When to Order Additional Testing

Supplemental testing (including blood tests, radiographic studies, or a spinal fluid examination) may be indicated in patients whose histories or examinations suggest secondary causes of headache. Any new headache (whether mild or severe) or substantial change in headache pattern should raise concern for possible secondary headache.

Red flags help determine which patients should receive additional testing to rule out secondary headache during an ED headache visit (Box 2.9). A helpful mnemonic to look for important red flags is SNOOP (Table 2.4). Neurological signs and symptoms are important red flags. Seizures should always prompt additional testing. A few patients with migraine with aura may sometimes have transient focal neurological symptoms, including limb weakness, hemisensory loss, diplopia, dysarthria, and confusion as part of their headache attacks; in most cases, however, unless focal neurological signs and symptoms or mental status changes are typical of the individual patient's attacks, these should serve as red flags to prompt additional testing. Other than rare hypnic headaches (short duration, night-time headaches, or "alarm-clock" headache; see Chap. 6), primary headaches hardly ever begin as new headaches in adults over age 50. For example, migraine begins most commonly in females between ages 20 and 24 and males between 15 and 19 [28]. In men and women, respectively, 82 and 84% of migraines begin before age 35 and 96 and 97% before age 50 [28]. Thus, adults over age 50 with any new headache – with or without any additional red flags – will need additional evaluations for secondary headache to rule out giant cell arteritis as well as primary and/or secondary malignancy.

> **Pearl for the practitioner:**
> Primary headaches rarely begin after age 50. Headache patients >50 years old with new onset headache should be evaluated for secondary headaches.

Box 2.9 Red Flags Suggesting the Need for Additional Work-up

- Trauma
- Fever
- Seizures
- New headache
- Change in previously stable headache pattern
- History of malignancy or HIV
- Neurological symptoms or signs
- Patient >50 years of age
- Time to peak headache intensity <5 min
- Severe pain over carotid arteries (may suggest vascular dissection)
- Headaches worse with coughing, sneezing, sexual relations, or Valsalva maneuver (e.g., bearing down to have a bowel movement)

Table 2.4 Use SNOOP to help identify patients with likely secondary headache

Mnemonic letter	Mnemonic words	Description
S	Systemic	Fever, weight loss, or decreased appetite often suggest systemic illness, including infection and malignancy
N	Neurological symptoms	Mental status changes, seizures, focal neurological signs or symptoms suggest possible brain pathology, e.g., CO poisoning, CVA, primary/secondary malignancy
O	Onset	New onset headaches that quickly reach peak intensity (thunderclap headaches) may occur in patients with subarachnoid hemorrhage or other secondary headaches, as well as cough or sex-related headaches
O	Older age	ED headaches are more likely to be secondary in older patients. Any new headache in patients >50 years old will need an evaluation for secondary headaches, including giant cell arteritis, acute glaucoma, and primary/secondary malignancy
P	Progressive course	Headache progression may signify a worsening underlying illness, such as space occupying lesions

CO carbon monoxide, CVA cerebrovascular accident

Box 2.10 American College of Emergency Physicians Recommendations About When to Scan an ED Headache Patient [29]

- New, abnormal findings on neuro exam (e.g., focal deficit or mental status/cognitive impairment)
- New, sudden onset, severe headache (thunderclap headache)
- New headache in patients with HIV/AIDs
- New headache in patient >50 years old

To Scan or Not to Scan?

Patients presenting with unusual or atypical headache histories or with headaches associated with red flags (Box 2.9) identified through SNOOP (Table 2.4) often need additional testing with neuroimaging. The American College of Emergency Physicians has published specific recommendations for imaging the ED headache patient (Box 2.10) [29].

Noncontrast CT is generally preferred over MRI for ED headache assessment to readily identify fractures, hemorrhage, and conditions associated with increased intracranial pressure. CT is particularly helpful for identifying serious pathology that requires urgent treatment. Some abnormalities, like acute, ischemic stroke, small hemorrhages, and posterior fossa pathology may not be readily identified on an initial CT scan. Obtaining a normal initial CT scan helps rule out many serious causes of secondary headaches, however, subsequent testing with MRI, vascular imaging (e.g., magnetic resonance angiography [MRA]), etc., may identify pathology. Patients needing further assessment with an MRI can often have this arranged as part of their follow-up care.

> **Pearl for the practitioner:**
> A noncontrast CT is the preferred initial imaging study for acute headache patients in the ED being evaluated for possible secondary headaches.

Patients with headaches associated with prominent neck pain may require additional imaging of the cervical spine or neck vasculature. Plain films of the cervical spine can show important degenerative changes as well as lytic or blastic lesions from primary or metastatic cancer. Asymptomatic, clinically insignificant abnormalities occur commonly in the cervical spine, especially around C5-6, with multilevel abnormalities in common [30]. Degenerative changes on cervical spine x-rays are most prevalent with increased age, with abnormalities seen in 70% of women and 95% of men between ages 60 and 65[31]. Patients with unilateral headaches and prominent neck pain may also need an evaluation like magnetic resonance angiography to rule out carotid dissection, which may occur after prolonged, abnormal neck posture, neck manipulation, or trauma.

Imaging in Patients with Suspected Cluster Headache

Patients diagnosed with most primary headaches, especially migraine and tension-type headache, typically do not need neuroimaging; however, a neuroimaging study should be performed for patients presenting with probable cluster-type headaches. Case reports of patients with short-lasting, trigeminal distribution headaches with ipsilateral autonomic features (including patients with presumptive diagnoses of cluster headache) who were subsequently diagnosed with secondary headaches were recently reviewed [32]. The most common secondary diagnoses were tumors (48% of cases; most commonly pituitary tumors [52% of all tumors]) and vascular lesions (39% of cases; most commonly carotid dissection [23% of vascular diagnoses], intracranial thrombosis [18%], intracerebral arteriovenous malformation [18%], and intracranial aneurysm [14%]). In many instances, these cases presented like typical cluster headache that responded to standard treatment. Because secondary headaches can mimic cluster headache, the authors recommended that all patients presenting with presumed cluster headache receive at least one imaging study (usually an MRI) before the diagnosis is firmly established. This is usually best arranged as an outpatient after discharge from the ED.

> **Pearl for the practitioner:**
> Secondary headaches can mimic cluster headache. Patients presenting with
> presumed cluster headache should have arrangements made for MRI testing
> to rule out secondary causes.

Spinal Fluid Examination

Patients without evidence of hemorrhage or increased intracranial pressure on brain
CT may need additional spinal fluid examination to detect small hemorrhages,
infection, and idiopathic intracranial hypertension. An imaging study of the head
should be performed prior to lumbar puncture when:

- Headache began after trauma;
- Increased intracranial pressure or hemorrhage is suspected;
- Seizure has occurred;
- Altered level of consciousness or focal neurological signs are present.

The reason that imaging should be performed prior to spinal tap in these circumstances is that if a mass is present and the intracranial pressure is elevated, the transient change in intracranial pressure associated with a spinal tap may result in brain
herniation.

Lumbar puncture is generally performed with the spine flexed by having the
patient lie in a curled, fetal position (lateral recumbent) to open the interspinous
spaces (Fig. 2.6). The needle is inserted in the space between the iliac crests, aiming
toward the navel. This position allows for accurate evaluation of opening and closing pressure. For obese patients, identification of landmarks is made easier by having the patient sit up and lean forward over a fixed bedside table to achieve this same
position (Fig. 2.7). While sitting makes retrieval of spinal fluid easier, opening and
closing pressure cannot accurately be assessed using this method.

Careful attention to technique can reduce the chance that postdural headaches
will occur. Box 2.11 describes characteristics that increase the risk of postdural
headache and tips on reducing postdural headache risk.

Expected normal results from a lumbar puncture in the lateral recumbent position
are shown in Table 2.5; opening pressure cannot be reliably measured when performed in the sitting position [33]. Abnormalities suggest additional testing. Opening
pressure can be elevated in patients with infections, tumors, SAH, and idiopathic
intracranial hypertension (previously called pseudotumor cerebri). Generally, studies
that should be ordered include cell count on tubes 1 and 4, gram stain and culture,
glucose and protein. Other studies, if indicated by history, may include Lyme titer,
the Venereal Disease Research Laboratory test (VDRL), viral, and/or fungal cultures.

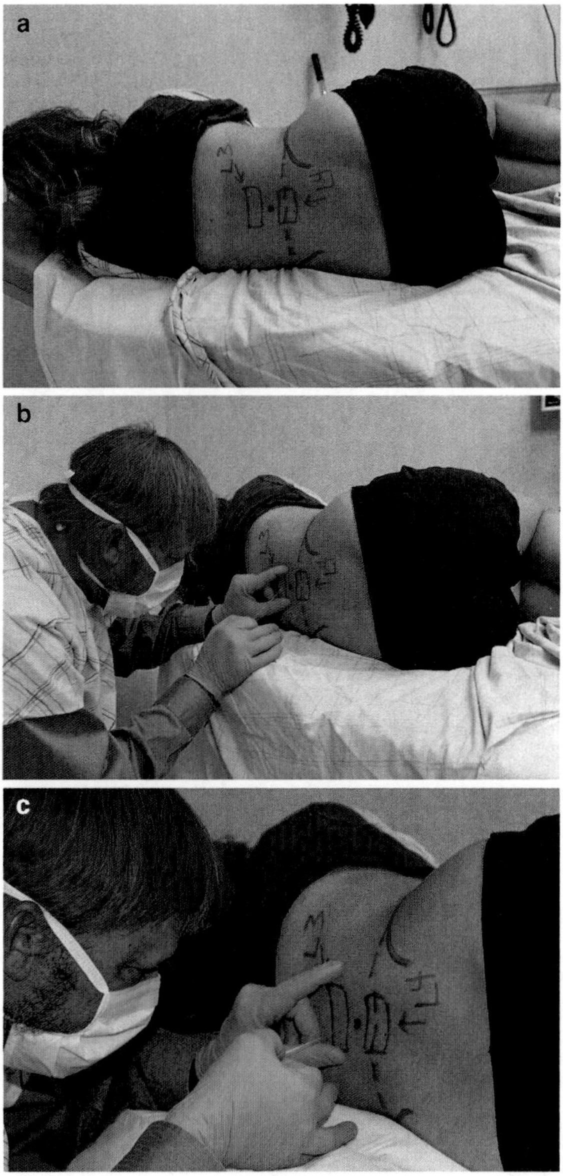

Fig. 2.6 Proper positioning
for a lumbar puncture.
(**a**) Patient positioning.
(**b**) Identifying landmarks.
(**c**) Needle placement

Fig. 2.7 Lumbar puncture in the leaning forward position (can be helpful in obese patients). (**a**) Patient positioning. (**b**) Needle placement

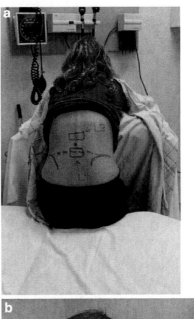

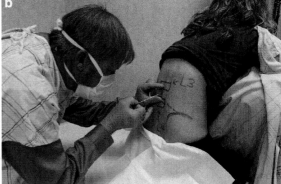

Pearl for the practitioner:
Usual studies that should be ordered for spinal fluid analysis include cell count on tubes 1 and 4, gram stain and culture, glucose, and protein. Other studies may be indicated in certain circumstances.

Red blood cells (RBCs) may not be detected in the spinal fluid until about 2 h or more after SAH. Spinal fluid examination is most sensitive about 12 h postbleed, when xanthochromia (yellowish fluid) is often seen. Xanthochromia results from RBC breakdown.

Box 2.11 Postdural Puncture Headache After Spinal Fluid Evaluation (Based on [40, 41])

- Recognizing patients at higher risk for developing postdural puncture headache

  - Age 20–30 years old
  - Female gender
  - Low body mass index
  - History of chronic headache
  - History of previous postdural puncture headache

- Reducing the occurrence of postdural puncture headache

  - While smaller gauge needles reduce postdural puncture headache, lumbar puncture requires a 22-gauge needle
  - Atraumatic needles (e.g., Sprotte and Whitacre) are preferred over cutting Quincke needles
  - If using a traumatic/cutting needle:
    - Orient the bevel to be parallel to the long axis of the spine rather than perpendicular to it
    - Reinsert the stylet prior to needle removal
    - When withdrawing the needle, maintain the orientation of the bevel parallel to the long axis of the spine to avoid dural tearing
  - Bed rest, hydration, patient position during the lumbar puncture (LP), volume of CSF removed are NOT linked to risk for postdural puncture headache

Xanthochromia can be assessed at the bedside by holding the test tube containing spinal fluid over a white piece of paper. A yellowish hue indicates that RBCs have broken down. Failure to identify xanthochromia, however, cannot be used to rule out hemorrhage. In an important study by Buruma and colleagues, a colorless supernatant was identified in 3 of 25 patients with documented intracranial hemorrhage [34]. Spectrophotometric screening of the supernatant at a wavelength of 415 nm for bilirubin effectively confirmed the presence of intracranial hemorrhage. Therefore, evaluation of the supernatant by the laboratory should be requested to help distinguish intracranial hemorrhage from traumatic tap. When spectrophotometry is not available, the American College of Emergency Physicians recommends having spinal fluid rapidly centrifuged and the supernatant compared against an identical tube containing clear water, with both tubes held together against a white background [35]. In this case, spinal fluid should be immediately hand-carried to the laboratory to facilitate rapid centrifugation. Although xanthochromia may not be visible during the first 12 h postbleed, this time of early bleed usually results in an abnormal CT and, when the CT is negative, large amounts of red blood cells in the spinal fluid [36]. Furthermore,

Table 2.5 Normal adult lumbar puncture results (based on [33])

Test	Normal value	Interpreting abnormal values
Appearance	Clear and colorless	Cloudy fluid may occur with increased white blood cells or protein. Brown to yellowish fluid may represent increased protein or bleeding >3 days previously. Reddish fluid may occur due to hemorrhage or traumatic spinal tap
Opening pressure in the lateral recumbent position	180 mmH$_2$O (200–250 mmH$_2$O in obese patient)	Both elevated and low blood pressures can be significant. Low pressures occur with spinal fluid leaks, while high pressure suggest elevated intracranial pressure such as seen with infections, subarachnoid hemorrhage, tumors, or idiopathic intracranial hypertension
White blood cells	0–5: mononuclear cells (lymphocytes and monocytes) 0: polymorphonuclear leukocytes	Increased white blood cells occur in patients with infection, inflammatory conditions, or malignancy
Glucose	65% of serum glucose <45 mg/dL is abnormal	High glucose occurs in patients with elevated serum glucose. Low glucose can occur in patients with hypoglycemia, as well as infection. CSF:blood glucose ratio ≤0.4 suggests bacterial meningitis [42]
Protein	≤50 mg/dL	Elevated protein may occur in patients with trauma, tumor, infection, inflammation, and diabetes

opening pressure is elevated in about two of three patients with SAH, while it should not be elevated in patients experiencing a traumatic tap [36].

Sending the first and last tubes of spinal fluid collected for cell count is often recommended to help determine if a traumatic tap occurred by showing RBC clearing in the latter tube. In general, patients with hemorrhage will not show a decrease in counts across tubes while those with traumatic taps will. Buruma and colleagues, however, showed that, while this distinction holds when looking at samples collected from a number of patients, the distinction is not sufficient when analyzing only an individual's sample of tubes [34]. In other words, monitoring reductions in RBCs across tubes cannot be used to confidently distinguish hemorrhage vs. traumatic tap.

> **Pearl for the practitioner:**
> Bedside inspection of spinal fluid for clearing of red coloring across tubes or xanthochromia, while often helpful, is inadequate to accurately rule out an intracranial hemorrhage. Spectrophotometric screening for bilirubin by the lab can help distinguish true hemorrhage from a traumatic tap.

According to recommendations from the American College of Emergency Physicians, a lumbar puncture and spinal fluid examination should be performed in patients with:

- A normal noncontrast CT;
- A presentation of sudden-onset, severe (thunderclap) headache or;
- A history or examination suggesting possible intracranial infection (e.g., meningitis) [29].

Additional testing (e.g., angiography) is not recommended in the ED for patients with thunderclap headache who have had a normal CT scan, normal opening pressure on lumbar puncture, and a normal spinal fluid analysis [29]. These patients are recommended to be symptomatically treated and discharged with close primary care follow-up. Depending on their history, these patients may be subsequently evaluated with noninvasive vascular testing (e.g., magnetic resonance angiography and venography or computerized tomographic angiography) of the head and neck vessels to rule out vascular pathology [37].

This recommendation from the American College of Emergency Physicians is supported by an important prospective study in which 592 patients presenting to two EDs with new onset, traumatic headache that reached maximal intensity in <1 h were evaluated with CT and spinal fluid examination [38]. Patients were then followed 6–36 months later to ensure that a diagnosis of SAH was not missed in the ED and later identified. In this cohort, SAH was diagnosed in the ED in 61 patients (55 through abnormal CT and 6 with abnormal spinal fluid). No additional cases were subsequently identified, supporting that the combination of CT and spinal fluid examination is appropriate and generally sufficient for diagnosing SAH.

Other Tests

Blood tests may be recommended in patients with symptoms or signs suggesting additional medical conditions or in patients >50 years old with a new headache to rule out giant cell arteritis (GCA; also called temporal arteritis) (Box 2.12 and Table 2.6). Both erythrocyte sedimentation rate (ESR) and C-reactive protein (CRP) have been recommended to screen for GCA. CRP rises in response to tissue injury earlier than ESR, suggesting that this might be a more sensitive screen in patients with new onset symptoms. A study evaluating inflammatory markers in 119 patients with biopsy proven GCA showed CRP to be a more sensitive diagnostic test than ESR (Fig. 2.8) [39]. An abnormal ESR was identified in 77% of patients, with an abnormal CRP in 98% ($P = 0.0003$). Also, ESR is less accurate in the setting of anemia. Patients with GCA may also report additional systemic symptoms, such as proximal muscle weakness/aching, fever, tongue/jaw claudication ("chewing or talking is tiring"), and/or subcutaneous painful cords (i.e., arteries) in the temples.

Table 2.6 Blood work to rule out giant cell arteritis (GCA)

Test	Normal adult values	Abnormalities suggesting GCA
CBC	WBC: 4500–11,000/mm³ Hemoglobin varies by gender • Males: 13.5–17.5 g/dL • Females: 12.0–16.0 g/dL Platelets: 150,000–400,000/mm³	Leukocytosis, anemia, or thrombocytosis
Erythrocyte sedimentation rate (ESR)	Normal ESR levels vary by age and gender [43] • For males: age × 0.5 • For females: (age × 0.5) + 5	Most patients with temporal arteritis have an ESR >80 mm/h; however, up to 20% of patients with GCA may have a normal or low ESR. Patients with anemia or blood dyscrasias, such as myelodysplasia, may have a normal ESR; rely on CRP for these patients
C-reactive protein (CRP)	<0.5 mg/dL Does not vary with age or gender	>2.45 mg/dL Abnormal CRP is more sensitive than ESR

WBC white blood cell

Box 2.12 Giant Cell Arteritis Symptoms

- New onset headache typically in adults >50 years old
- Headache
- Scalp sensitivity
- Fever
- Malaise and fatigue
- Muscle aches
- Jaw pain, especially with chewing
- Vision changes

Putting It All Together

Figure 2.9 summarizes how to decide which specific tests should be considered for each individual headache patient in the ED. Most patients in the ED will have a primary headache and additional testing beyond a history and physical examination will not be necessary. Additional testing is most beneficial to determine the specific cause of possible secondary headaches.

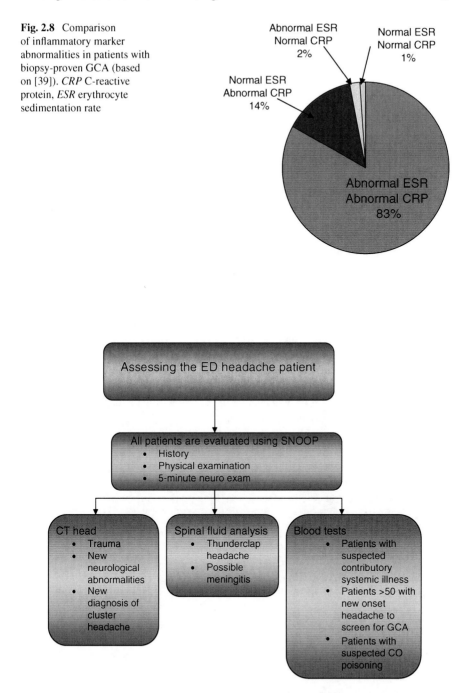

Fig. 2.8 Comparison of inflammatory marker abnormalities in patients with biopsy-proven GCA (based on [39]). *CRP* C-reactive protein, *ESR* erythrocyte sedimentation rate

Fig. 2.9 History and examination are required in all patients, while additional testing is generally limited to patients with warning symptoms or signs that suggest possible secondary headache. *CO* carbon monoxide, *CT* computed tomography, *GCA* giant cell arteritis

Online Resources for Patient Assessment

- Detailed neurological examination
  - http://www.neuroexam.com
- Lumbar puncture
  - Instructional video available through the New England Journal of Medicine at http://www.nejm.org
- Fundoscopic examination, which includes the use of a Panoptic fundoscope
  - http://stanford25.wordpress.com

Summary

- The primary goal for headache evaluation in the ED is to rule out dangerous secondary headaches. Determining the specific type of primary headache is less important. Patients determined to have a probable primary headache do not need to have additional evaluations to determine the specific type of primary headache during their ED visit. Secondary headaches will be covered in more detail in Chap. 3.
- Most patients with a primary headache in the ED will have migraine, which can be preliminarily screened for using the three-item ID-Migraine questionnaire once secondary causes of headache have been considered.
- A series of six essential headache questions can be used to categorize patients as those with a problematic chronic primary headache or a headache needing further evaluation as a possible secondary headache.
- Sudden onset, new, severe headaches reaching peak intensity within 5 min (thunderclap headache) should be evaluated for possible SAH.
- Careful observation during history taking allows an effective neurological assessment to be condensed into about 5 min.
- Neuroimaging, spinal fluid examination, and blood work are generally best reserved for patients with likely secondary headaches suggesting pathology that requires urgent assessment.

References

1. Friedman BW, Hochberg ML, Esses D, et al. Applying the International Classification of Headache Disorders to the emergency department: an assessment of reproducibility and the frequency with which a unique diagnosis can be assigned to every acute headache presentation. Ann Emerg Med. 2007;49:409–19.

2. Breen DP, Duncan CW, Pope AE, Gray AJ, Salman RA. Emergency department evaluation of sudden severe headache. Q J Med. 2008;101:435–43.
3. Matharu MS, Schwedt TJ, Dodick DW. Thunderclap headache: an approach to a neurologic emergency. Curr Neruol Neurosci Rep. 2007;7:101–9.
4. Eross E, Dodick D, Eross M. The sinus, allergy, migraine study. Headache. 2007;47:213–24.
5. Obermann M, Yoon MS, Dommes P, et al. Prevalence of trigeminal autonomic symptoms in migraine: a population-based study. Cephalalgia. 2007;27:504–9.
6. Schreiber CP, Hutchinson S, Webster CJ, et al. Prevalence of migraine in patients with a history of self-reported or physician-diagnosed "sinus" headache. Arch Intern Med. 2004;164: 1769–72.
7. Lipton RB, Dodick D, Sadovsky R, et al. A self-administered screener for migraine in primary care: the ID Migraine™ validation study. Neurology. 2003;61:375–82.
8. Mostardini C, d'Agostino VC, Dugoni DE, Cerbo R. A possible role of ID-Migraine in the emergency department: study of an emergency department out-patient population. Cephalalgia. 2009;29:1326–30.
9. Bigal ME, Ashina S, Burstein R, et al. Prevalence and characteristics of allodynia in headache sufferers: a population study. Neurology. 2008;70:1525–33.
10. Tietjen GE, Brandes JL, Peterlin BL, et al. Allodynia in migraine: association with comorbid pain conditions. Headache. 2009;49:1333–44.
11. Lovati C, D'Amico D, Bertora P. Allodynia in migraine: frequent random association or unavoidable consequence? Exp Rev Neurother. 2009;9:395–408.
12. Madden T, Rosen N, Young W. Exploring home allodynia testing for future clinical and scientific uses. Headache. 2009;49:132–4.
13. Friedman B, Bijur P, Greenwalk P, Lipton R, Gallagher EJ. Clinical significance of brush allodynia in emergency patients with migraine. Headache. 2009;49:31–5.
14. Burstein R, Jakubowski M. Analgesic triptan action in an animal model of intracranial pain: a race against the development of central sensitization. Ann Neurol. 2004;55:27–36.
15. Burstein R, Collins B, Jakubowski M. Defeating migraine pain with triptans: a race against the development of cutaneous allodynia. Ann Neurol. 2004;55:19–26.
16. Cady RK, Freitag FG, Mathew NT, et al. Allodynia-associated symptoms, pain intensity and time to treatment: predicting treatment response in acute migraine intervention. Headache. 2009;49:350–63.
17. Schoenen J, De Klippel N, Giurgea S, et al. Almotriptan and its combination with aceclofenac for migraine attacks: a study of efficacy and the influence of auto-evaluated brush allodynia. Cephalalgia. 2008;28:1095–105.
18. Kalita J, Yadav RK, Misra UK. A comparison of migraine patients with and without allodynic symptoms. Clin J Pain. 2009;25:696–8.
19. Pozo-Rosich P, Oshinsky ML. Dihydroergotamine (DHE) blocks the induction of central sensitization in the trigeminal nucleus caudalis [abstract]. Neurology. 2005;64:A151.
20. Silberstein SD, Young WB, Hopkins MM, et al. Dihydroergotamine for early and late treatment of migraine with cutaneous allodynia: an open-label pilot trial. Headache. 2007;47:878–85.
21. Ibañez J, Arikan F, Pedraza S, et al. Reliability of clinical guidelines in the detection of patients at risk following mild head injury: results of a prospective study. J Neurosurg. 2004;100:825–34.
22. Saboori M, Ahmadi J, Farajzadegan Z. Indications for brain CT scan in patients with minor head injury. Clin Neurol Neurosurg. 2007;109:399–405.
23. Holm L, Cassidy JD, Carroll LJ, Borg J. Summary of the WHO Collaborating Centre for neurotrauma task force on mild traumatic brain injury. J Rehabil Med. 2005;27:137–41.
24. Hylleraas S, Davidsen EM, Benth JS, Gulbrandsen P, Dietrichs E. The usefulness of testing head and neck muscle tenderness and neck mobility in acute headache patients. Funct Neurol. 2010;25:27–31.
25. Barbanti P, Aurilia C, Egeo G, Fofi L. Hypertension as a risk factor for migraine chronification. Neurol Sci. 2010;31 Suppl 1:S41–3.
26. Gippono S, Venturelli E, Rao R, Liberini P, Padovani A. Hypertension is a factor associated with chronic daily headache. Neurol Sci. 2010;31 Suppl 1:S171–3.

27. Friedman BW, Grosberg BM. Diagnosis and management of the primary headache disorders in the emergency department setting. Emerg Med Clin N Am. 2009;27:71.
28. Stewart WF, Wood C, Reed ML, et al. Cumulative lifetime migraine incidence in women and men. Cephalalgia. 2008;28:1170–8.
29. Edlow JA, Panagos PD, Godwin SA, Thomas TL, Decker WW. American College of Emergency Physician. Clinical policy: critical issues in the evaluation and management of adult patients presenting to the emergency department with acute headache. Ann Emerg Med. 2008;52:407–36.
30. Gore DR. Roentgenographic findings in the cervical spine in asymptomatic persons. A ten-year follow-up. Spine. 2001;26:2463–6.
31. Gore DR, Sepic SB, Gardner GM. Roentgenographic findings of the cervical spine in asymptomatic people. Spine. 1986;11(6):521–4.
32. Wilbrink LA, Perrari MD, Kruit MC, Haan J. Neuroimaging in trigeminal autonomic cephalalgias: when, how, and of what? Curr Opin Neurol. 2009;22:247–53.
33. Roos KL. Lumbar puncture. Semin Neurol. 2003;23:105–14.
34. Buruma OJ, Janson HL, Den Bergh FA, Bots GT. Bloodstained cerebrospinal fluid: traumatic puncture or haemorrhage? J Neurol Neurosurg Psychiatry. 1981;44:144–7.
35. Edlow JA, Panagos PD, Godwin SA, Thomas TL, Decker WW. Clinical policy: critical issues in the evaluation and management of adult patients presenting to the emergency department with acute headache. Ann Emerg Med. 2008;52:407–36.
36. Edlow JA, Malek AM, Ogilvy CS. Aneurysmal subarachnoid hemorrhage: update for emergency physicians. J Emerg Med. 2008;34:237–51.
37. Ju YS, Schwedt TJ. Abrupt-onset severe headaches. Semin Neurol. 2010;30:192–200.
38. Perry JJ, Spacke A, Forbes M, et al. Is the combination of negative computed tomography result and negative lumbar puncture result sufficient to rule out subarachnoid hemorrhage? Ann Emerg Med. 2008;51:707–13.
39. Parikh M, Miller NR, Lee AG, et al. Prevalence of a normal C-reactive protein with an elevated erythrocyte sedimentation rate in biopsy-proven giant cell arteritis. Ophthalmology. 2006;113:1842–5.
40. Bezov D, Ashina S, Lipton R. Post-dural puncture headache: part I. Diagnosis, epidemiology, etiology, and pathophysiology. Headache. 2010;50:1144–52.
41. Bezov D, Ashina S, Lipton R. Post-dural puncture headache: part II. Prevention, management, and prognosis. Headache. 2010;50:1482–98.
42. Strauss SE, Thorpe KE, Holroyd-Leduc J. How do I perform a lumbar puncture and analyze the results to diagnose bacterial meningitis? JAMA. 2006;296:2012–22.
43. Miller A, Green M, Robinson D. Simple rule for calculating normal erythrocyte sedimentation rate. Br Med J (Clin Res Ed). 1983;286:266.

Chapter 3
Secondary Headaches

Key Chapter Points

- Possible secondary headaches need to be considered initially for all patients presenting to the ED with acute headache. (See Chapter 2 for assessment strategies.)
- Always consider trauma as a possible cause of acute headache.
- Brain injury severity, demographic features, and examination findings help determines the need for additional testing in patients with headache after trauma.
- Headache due to arterial dissection in the neck may occur after seemingly insignificant neck trauma (e.g., whiplash injury, spinal manipulation, or prolonged abnormal posture).
- Meningitis may be considered in patients with non-traumatic headache plus fever, neck stiffness, or altered mental status.
- Idiopathic intracranial hypertension may be considered in obese females with headache, transient visual loss, and papilledema. Imaging studies will fail to show intracranial mass lesions in these patients.
- Thunderclap headaches must always be evaluated fully before the diagnosis of primary thunderclap headache is assigned.

Keywords Carotid dissection • Concussion • Meningitis • Idiopathic intracranial hypertension • Thunderclap headache • Trauma

Ruling out secondary headaches is a major responsibility of the emergency department (ED) staff – even though most patients coming to the ED with a complaint of headache will have a benign, primary headache (see Chap. 1). Patients categorized as having a headache PLUS other symptoms or signs OR headache in patients with known and likely contributory medical illnesses (using the six essential ED headache questions in Chap. 2) should be carefully evaluated for possible secondary headaches (Table 3.1). In addition, new headaches occurring in patients >50 years old will require more extensive evaluation for secondary headache causes.

D.A. Marcus and P.A. Bain, *Practical Assessment and Treatment of the Patient*   53
with Headaches in the Emergency Department and Urgent Care Clinic,
DOI 10.1007/978-1-4614-0002-8_3, © Springer Science+Business Media, LLC 2011

Table 3.1 Secondary headache diagnoses

Disease categories	Examples
Trauma	Concussion
	Cervicocranial artery dissection
Infection	Systemic infection
	Sinusitis
	Meningitis
	Encephalitis
Vascular disease	Subarachnoid hemorrhage
	Stroke
	Cervicocranial artery dissection
	Cerebral venous and dural sinus thrombosis
	Giant cell (temporal) arteritis
	Hypertension
Toxic exposures	Carbon monoxide poisoning
Intracranial mass lesions	Tumor
	Abscess
	Hematoma
	Third ventricle colloid cyst
Eye disease	Acute narrow angle glaucoma
Other	Idiopathic intracranial hypertension (pseudotumor cerebri)

Although patients are often concerned about brain tumor as the cause for their headache, headaches related to brain tumors are usually mild and infrequently result in an ED visit. Most brain tumors result in other neurological abnormalities, e.g., seizure, cognitive change, or focal deficits, before patients complain of headache (Fig. 3.1).

> **Pearl for the practitioner:**
> A diagnosis of secondary headache is most likely in patients with:
>
> - Headache PLUS other symptoms or signs
> - Headache in patients with known and likely contributory medical illnesses
> - New headaches occurring in adults over 50 years old, with risk increasing with age

Important, more common secondary headaches discussed in this chapter include both traumatic and nontraumatic headaches:

- Traumatic headaches

  - Mild brain injury with concussion
  - Cervicocranial artery dissection

- Nontraumatic headaches

  - Subarachnoid hemorrhage (SAH)
  - Cough, sexual activity related, and exertional headaches

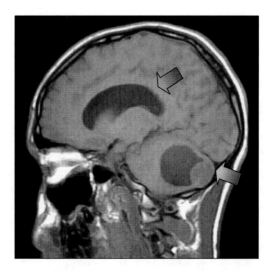

Fig. 3.1 Intracranial mass lesion with hydrocephalus. Patients with intracranial mass lesions generally do not complain of substantial headaches until the lesions are quite large, such as the one seen here in the T-1 weighted magnetic resonance image. This saggital image of the head shows a large cystic tumor in the cerebellum (lower *yellow arrow*) that is blocking cerebrospinal fluid outflow from the lateral ventricles (upper *blue arrow*) with resultant hydrocephalus (image courtesy of Clayton A. Wiley, MD)

- Meningitis
- Cerebral venous thrombosis
- Idiopathic intracranial hypertension (previously called pseudotumor cerebri)
- Giant cell arteritis
- Anginal equivalent headaches
- CO poisoning
- Acute glaucoma

Traumatic Headache

Patients presenting to the ED for evaluation of headache after trauma will need a careful history and examination to determine the likely extent of the trauma. The American Congress of Rehabilitation Medicine Special Interest Group on Mild Traumatic Brain Injury Patients and American College of Emergency Physicians have published criteria for diagnosing a concussion and determining whether that concussion represents a mild or more severe brain injury (Table 3.2) [1, 2]. Patients experiencing symptoms that are more severe than those constituting a mild traumatic brain injury will need neck x-rays and a noncontrast computed tomography (CT). Recommendations for obtaining a noncontrast head CT for patients with mild brain injury are given in Table 3.3.

Table 3.2 Diagnosing mild brain injury [1, 2]

A concussion has occurred when *any* of the following is reported:	A concussion is considered a mild traumatic brain injury with *all* of the following:
• Feeling dazed or confused after the head injury • "Seeing stars" • "Getting the wind knocked out" • Losing consciousness for any amount of time • Losing memory for the time immediately before or after the head injury	• Nonpenetrating head trauma • Patient presents to ED within 24 h of injury • Glasgow Coma Scale score 14–15 (see Chap. 2) • Any loss of consciousness lasting ≤30 min • Any amnesia involving <24 h of time lost

Table 3.3 American College of Emergency Physicians recommendations for neuroimaging in patients ≥16 years old with mild traumatic brain injury (based on [2])

A noncontrast brain CT should be obtained in the ED when:	
Mild traumatic brain injury WITH loss of consciousness or post-trauma amnesia. Obtain imaging study when any one of the following is present:	Mild traumatic brain injury with NO loss of consciousness or post-trauma amnesia. Obtain imaging study when any one of the following is present:

• Historical features
  – Age >60 years
  – Bleeding disorder
  – Drug or alcohol intoxication
• Symptoms
  – Headache
  – Vomiting
  – Seizure
• Signs
  – Physical evidence of trauma about the clavicle
  – Short-term memory loss
  – Focal neurological deficits
  – GCS score <15
	• Historical features
	  – Age ≥65 years
	  – Bleeding disorder
	  – Dangerous mechanism of injury (e.g., ejected from motor vehicle, motor vehicle-pedestrian accident, fall >3 feet or five steps)
	• Symptoms
	  – Severe headache
	  – Vomiting
	• Signs
	  – Physical evidence of skull fracture
	  – Focal neurological deficits
	  – GCS score <15

GCS Glasgow Coma Scale

According to the American College of Emergency Physicians, patients ≥16 years old with mild traumatic brain injury (Table 3.2) may be discharged from the ED with observation for symptom worsening at home if:

• They have no additional worrisome symptoms, e.g., focal neurological deficits, cognitive impairment, vomiting;
• They have a normal neurological examination;
• They had a normal noncontrast CT of the head;
• They have no history of coagulopathy or previous neurosurgical procedure.

These patients will need to be provided with information about postconcussive symptoms at the time of discharge (Box 3.1).

Box 3.1 Patient Instructions After Concussion

What Is a Concussion?

A concussion is a mild brain injury caused by trauma to the head. When you have a concussion, you may have some symptoms right away, like feeling dazed, getting a headache, or getting knocked out. You may also develop other symptoms that you may not notice for several days after the concussion:

- Difficulty with concentration or memory
- Feeling irritable, sad, or extra-emotional
- Having a headache
- Feeling dizzy or off balance
- Having a change in your usual sleep pattern

These symptoms occur quite commonly in people after a concussion and usually go away over days to months.

How Can I Get Better Faster?

The best way to help your brain heal after a concussion is to let it rest. So get lots of rest and sleep and avoid activities that are either physically or mentally taxing. Reading may be especially tiring. Even playing games may be too much work for your brain. Avoid making important decisions if you feel mentally cloudy or are having problems concentrating or remembering things. Make sure your doctor has cleared you to drive before getting behind the wheel. Be sure to talk to your doctor to see if you should consider taking time off from school or work.

It's also important to avoid reinjuring your brain. When you have a concussion, your brain doesn't react as quickly while it's healing – this puts you at increased risk for having another concussion. So avoid activities that might result in falls or injury. You should also avoid drinking alcohol at this time.

When Can I Get Back in the Game?

You will need to wait until you feel all better before starting to play sports again. Returning to your sport too early will likely make you feel worse, slow your recovery, and put you at risk for added injuries. This isn't good for you or your team. Once you feel all better – which usually takes only a few days or weeks – your coach should have you gradually return to your sport. You will need to start with very light activities. Your coach can advance your activity level no faster than once every day. It will take a minimum of 1 full week to get from first starting to return with light activities to being in the game.

(continued)

Box 3.1 (continued)

When Should I Call the Doctor or Go Back to the Emergency Room?

Let your doctor know if any of your symptoms is getting worse, doesn't go away, or is causing substantial disability.

Go to the hospital right away if you start having problems with:

- Seizures
- Repeated vomiting
- Worsening of your headache
- Problems staying awake or alert
- Increased confusion
- Problems with your vision
- Problems that concern you, your family, or your friends

After you've had a concussion, it's sometimes hard to see how you're doing. Your family and friends can be good judges about whether you're acting differently than normal.

Postconcussion Activity Restrictions

Case 1

Tyler is a 17-year-old high school junior who is the starting pitcher for his baseball team. During last night's game, Tyler was hit in the head with a ball during the eighth inning. When he was hit, he fell over and he didn't respond to his team-mates until his coach ran across the field. Tyler was slightly disoriented, complained about feeling dizzy, and thought he was going to throw up. Tyler was sent to the ED where his neurological examination and head CT were normal. Tyler returned to play the next night. He told the coach he felt okay before the game, but after three innings, his head was pounding and he felt very dizzy again. His mother returned to the ED wondering if the doctor's missed something their first visit. "Tyler was basically fine this morning, but now his headache and dizziness are so much worse. Did something else happen besides just a concussion?"

Tyler experienced a concussion with mild brain injury. His aggravation of symptoms after resuming activities following a concussion is not unusual. Patients and their families need to understand that a concussion signifies trauma to the brain. This injury requires healing time and patients should never feel like "it's just a concussion" so no additional care is needed. Providing instructions about appropriate brain rest after concussion is essential to speed patient recovery and avoid over-exertion with symptomatic aggravation and additional ED visits.

After a concussion, it is essential that the patient allows for time to recover. This requires both physical and cognitive rest. Engaging in either physical exertion or mentally taxing activities – e.g., work, school, playing games, and driving – will often aggravate or trigger symptoms and delay recovery. When cognitive deficits occur, patients may need to complete neuropsychological testing to determine when they are ready to return to work.

Nonprofessional athletes experiencing a sport-related concussion should discontinue their sport until an appropriate time for recovery has lapsed and they have successfully completed a gradual return of activities (Table 3.4) [3]. Computerized neurocognitive testing is often used by sports medicine physicians and trainers for determining when athletes can return to their previous activities following a concussion. Information on the commonly used Immediate Postconcussion Assessment and Cognitive Testing (ImPACT) can be found online at http://www.impacttest.com/. Reliance on standardized testing results, however, requires caution as some experts argue that baseline testing has not been shown to reduce concussion risk and testing results after injury may result in premature return to play [4]. A survey of sports medicine professionals at 399 high school and university athletic programs

Table 3.4 Graduated return to play protocol for the amateur or student athlete (based on [3])

Stage of recovery	Recommended activity level
Immediate postconcussion period through time when any symptoms are still present	No sports participation. Patient needs physical and cognitive rest, avoiding activities that require physical exertion (e.g., exercise) or are mentally taxing (e.g., work, schoolwork, videogames, text messaging, driving, etc.)
After the patient is symptom-free, he/she may start light aerobic exercise	Low-intensity walking, swimming, or stationary bicycling. Keep heart rate to <70% of maximum predicted rate. Resistance training is NOT permitted
If the patient has no aggravation of symptoms after 24 h with light aerobic exercise, he/she may advance to a sport-specific activity	For example, running or skating drills where no head impact or contact is anticipated
If the patient has no aggravation of symptoms after 24 h with a sport-specific activity, he/she may advance to noncontact training drills	More complex training drills may be started, e.g., passing drills where no head impact or contact is anticipated
If the patient has no aggravation of symptoms after 24 h with noncontact training drills, he/she may advance to full contact practice	Medical clearance should be obtained prior to resuming full contact sport
If the patient has no aggravation of symptoms after 24 h with full contact practice, he/she may return to play	Normal game play, as tolerated

After becoming asymptomatic, the athlete needs to spend at least 1 additional day at each exercise stage before advancing to the next level. He/she should only advance if the exercise is tolerated with NO aggravation of postconcussion symptoms. If symptoms are aggravated, the athlete should return to the previously tolerated level of activity until comfortable and then reinitiate the graduated return to play protocol, as tolerated

using ImPACT testing found that following a concussion, 96% would not return a symptomatic athlete to play, even if neurocognitive testing scores were at baseline levels; 87% would hold an asymptomatic player back from play due to abnormal testing, while 10% would allow an asymptomatic player with worsened neurocognitive testing to return to play [5].

> *Pearl for the practitioner:*
> Patients need to be treated with mental and physical rest after a concussion to facilitate recovery. Return to sports should occur only after symptoms have resolved and a gradual return to play has been successfully completed. The decision to return to play may be assisted by using standardized neurocognitive testing.

> *Pearl for the practitioner:*
> Online resources and guidelines for mild traumatic brain injury can be found at
>
> - The Centers for Disease Control and Prevention web site: http://www.cdc.gov/traumaticbraininjury/
> - The American Academy of Neurology web site: http://www.aan.com/
> - The American Academy of Orthopaedic Surgeons web site: http://www.aaos.org/
> - The American Orthopaedic Society for Sports Medicine web site: http://www.sportsmed.org
> - The American Medical Society for Sports Medicine web site: http://www.amssm.org/

Cervicocranial Artery Dissection

Cervicocranial arterial dissection is relatively uncommon, although a leading cause of stroke in young adults. Dissection most commonly affects the extracranial internal carotid or vertebral arteries [6]. Most cases occur after trauma to the head or neck (Box 3.2) [7]. Dissection may occur from direct blows to the neck, as well as injuries that cause neck hyperextension or rotation that stretches vessels. Carotid dissections have been reported with a variety of sports, including baseball, boxing, cycling, football, hockey, scuba diving, skating, skiing, softball, Taekwondo, and weightlifting [8]. In some cases, trauma may appear minor, such as neck manipulation or prolonged abnormal neck posture. Interestingly, a literature review found more cases of cervical artery dissection attributed to chiropractic manipulation than to motor vehicle accidents [9]. Another contributing factor in some cases of dissection, fibromuscular dysplasia, occurs in about 15% of cases of spontaneous, nontraumatic dissection [10].

Box 3.2 Examples of Precipitating Trauma for Cervicocranial Artery Dissection

- Direct blow to the neck
- Chiropractic manipulation
- Whiplash injury
- Yoga
- Painting a ceiling
- Coughing
- Sneezing
- Vomiting
- Neck extension related to general anesthesia or resuscitation
- Weight lifting

Pearl for the practitioner:
Cervicocranial arterial dissection may occur after major or seemingly minor trauma to the head or neck. Usually, injury occurs following direct trauma to the neck or hyperextension or rotation injuries.

Cervicocranial arterial dissection most commonly results in ischemic stroke or SAH (Table 3.5). Headache involving the eye, face, and ear on the side of the dissection occurs in 74% of cases of cervicocranial arterial dissections [11], though usually not as an isolated symptom. A retrospective review of 73 cases of nontraumatic dissection showed the most typical presentations to be ischemic stroke (55%) and SAH (30%) [12]. Only four patients presented with headache (5%), located on the side of the dissection in each case. Among the 40 patients presenting with an ischemic stroke, 55% had an accompanying headache and/or neck pain lateralized to the side of the dissection. All patients presenting with a SAH had a headache. Mean age among these patients was 45.

Pearl for the practitioner:
Patients with cervicocranial arterial dissection usually report ipsilateral headache, although headache is rarely the only symptom reported.

Patients with suspected cervicocranial arterial dissection need evaluation with vascular imaging. Noninvasive testing with magnetic resonance imaging and angiography or computed tomography angiography may confirm the diagnosis, although

Table 3.5 Common symptoms in patients with cervicocranial arterial dissection

Carotid artery	Vertebral artery
Cerebral ischemia	Ataxia
Monocular blindness	Diplopia
Partial Horner's (ptosis and miosis) with internal carotid dissection	Dizziness and vertigo
	Dysarthria
Sweating loss (anhidrosis) on one side of the face with external carotid dissection	Lateral medullary stroke or Wallenberg's syndrome (numbness on one side of the face and the opposite side of the body, Horner's, dysphasia, vertigo; weakness on one side of the face and the opposite side of the body and uncontrolled hiccups may also occur)

computed tomography angiography is often more sensitive in identifying carotid rather than vertebral dissection [13]. Typical imaging and pathology findings are shown in Fig. 3.2.

Nontraumatic Headache

Sudden Onset, Severe, Nontraumatic Headache

Abrupt onset of the "worst headache of my life" is often linked to concerns for a diagnosis of SAH, often from a leaking cerebral aneurysm. A sudden onset headache that reaches peak severity in seconds or minutes is often called a "thunderclap" headache. While thunderclap headaches may signify important underlying pathology, they may also occur as a benign, primary headache disorder. The diagnosis, however, of primary thunderclap headache can only be made if more ominous causes of thunderclap headache can be ruled out, which typically requires a physical examination, imaging study, and spinal fluid analysis (see Chap. 2).

> **Pearl for the practitioner:**
> Abrupt onset headache reaching maximum intensity in ≤5 min is called a "thunderclap" headache. Appropriate workup for thunderclap headache includes brain imaging and spinal fluid analysis. Other testing, such as angiography, may also be needed.

Fig. 3.2 (continued) neck bones, the vertebral artery is usually secluded from traumatic disruption. (**b**) Pathology in a patient with trauma to the vertebral artery. Cross section of the vertebral artery from a trauma patient. The artery wall is thickened and the lumen compressed secondary to repeated trauma to a developmentally displaced vessel. Trauma to the vessel wall led to abnormal blood flow and eventually a lethal stroke

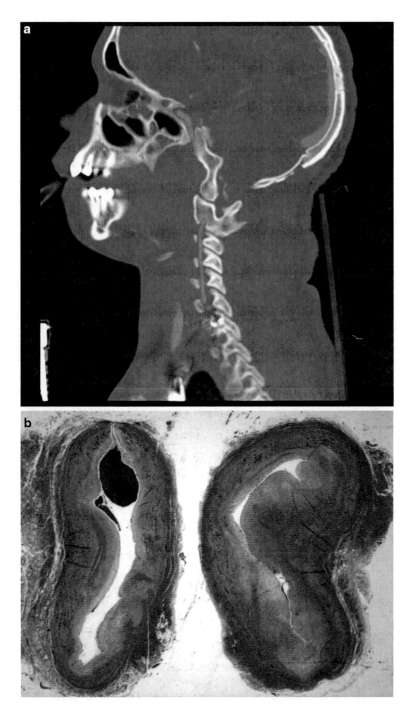

Fig. 3.2 Vertebral artery dissection (images courtesy of Clayton A. Wiley, MD, PhD). (**a**) Computed tomography, saggital view. This saggital scan of the head and neck shows one of the verte-bral arteries coursing up through the neck inside the vertebral column. Protected within the

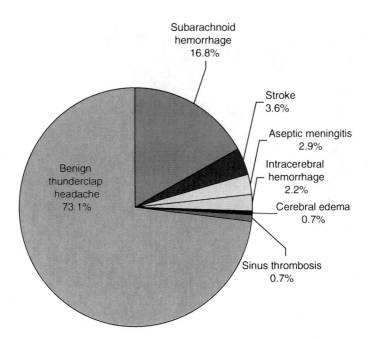

Subarachnoid
hemorrhage
16.8%

Stroke
3.6%

Aseptic meningitis
2.9%

Intracerebral
hemorrhage
2.2%

Benign
thunderclap
headache
73.1%

Cerebral edema
0.7%

Sinus thrombosis
0.7%

Fig. 3.3 Diagnoses assigned to consecutive ED patients seen for sudden onset headache (based on [15])

Unfortunately, characteristic features touted as clinical hallmarks of SAH, such as very rapid onset of pain, experiencing an unusually severe or "the worst" headache, and having transient focal symptoms, have not been shown to distinguish SAH from benign thunderclap headache [14]. Thunderclap headache in the ED was evaluated in a 31-month study in Sweden [15]. All patients were evaluated in the ED with a CT scan and follow-up spinal tap if a hemorrhage was not diagnosed on the CT scan. A total of 137 patients were evaluated, with SAH diagnosed in 23 patients (17%; Fig. 3.3). CT scan was normal in five patients who were subsequently diagnosed with SAH through spinal fluid testing. Patients with SAH were more likely to be older (56 years vs. 39 years, $P=0.0002$). Patients with SAH were also more likely to report occipital location pain ($P=0.03$), nausea ($P=0.007$), neck stiffness ($P<0.0001$), and impaired consciousness ($P=0.03$). Interestingly, a personal or family history of migraine was similar between patients with and without SAH. Patients without SAH were followed for up to 1 year. Recurrent attacks of thunderclap headaches occurred in 24% of those without SAH. This study highlights that, while benign headache is the most common diagnosis among patients presenting with a sudden onset, severe headache, clinical features fail to predict which patients will have serious SAH or other pathological secondary headaches. Therefore, all patients presenting with their first episode of thunderclap headache should be evaluated with a thorough history and physical examination, along with CT *AND* spinal fluid testing, when CT testing is negative, to rule out hemorrhage, infarction, or infection. Additional testing with angiography should generally be reserved for patients with symptoms or physical examination signs suggesting pathology or abnormal CT or spinal fluid testing.

> **Pearl for the practitioner:**
> Thunderclap headache is more likely to be caused by SAH when patients
>
> - Are older
> - Report occipital pain
> - Have nausea
> - Report neck stiffness
> - Experienced impaired consciousness

Subarachnoid Hemorrhage

SAH is a neurosurgical emergency as bleeding that occurs without trauma usually occurs from extravasation of blood from aneurysms or other vascular malformations. Risk factors and a differential diagnosis are shown in Boxes 3.3 and 3.4.

ED doctors are usually quite adept at identifying SAH and most patients with SAH will be identified before the diagnosis is confirmed through testing, based on abnormalities in the history and physical examination (Table 3.6). Evaluation typically includes imaging studies and a spinal fluid examination (Table 3.7). In an interesting study, ED physicians evaluated 747 headache patients, 77% of whom reported this was their "worst headache" [16]. SAH was eventually diagnosed in 50 of these patients. Although doctors were uncomfortable with not conducting additional testing to rule out a diagnosis for 75% of cases, they did a good job at clinically identifying who were likely to have a SAH before testing was conducted. Only three patients that the doctors thought had a relatively low likelihood of having a SAH were diagnosed with SAH after CT/spinal fluid assessment.

> **Pearl for the practitioner:**
> The prevalence of subarachnoid hemorrhage in an ED patient with sudden onset headache and a normal neurological exam is about 15% (based on [35]).

Perry and colleagues developed three series of questions to help identify neurologically intact patients at high risk for having SAH [17]. They identified 13 historical and 3 examination variables that reliably predicted patients with SAH (Table 3.8). Patients with sudden onset headache in whom SAH suspected will require a non-contrast CT scan and, if negative, spinal fluid analysis, even when neurological examination is normal.

The most difficult patients to diagnose are those with atypical histories or a previous chronic headache. It is, therefore, imperative for ED physicians to carfully review important signs and symptoms with patients and their families upon

Box 3.3 Risk Factors for SAH

- Postmenopausal woman
- Race and ethnicity

  - African
  - Asian
  - Hispanic

- Hypertension
- Inherited connective tissue disorders

  - Polycystic kidney disease
  - Ehlers–Danlos syndrome

- Substance abusers

  - Alcohol
  - Nicotine
  - Cocaine

- Trauma
- Family history of SAH in first-degree relative

Box 3.4 Differential Diagnosis for SAH

- Migraine
- Infection (meningitis, encephalitis)
- Giant cell arteritis
- Cerebral venous thrombosis
- Other cerebral hemorrhage or ischemia
- Craniocervical dissection

discharge that should prompt urgent reevaluation in the ED. These instructions should be provided in writing for patients and families (see Chap. 9). SAH is treated with medical stabilization and urgent neurosurgical consultation.

Cough, Sexual Activity Related, and Exertional Headaches

Headaches occurring in relationship to cough, physical exertion, or sexual activity may be caused by primary (see Chap. 1) or secondary headaches (e.g., cerebral aneurysm rupture or cerebral artery dissection). In an interesting study, 97 patients with headache occurring during Valsalva maneuvers, physical exertion, or sexual activity were followed prospectively for 1 year [18]. A total of 53 patients were

Table 3.6 Typical SAH characteristics

Category	Description
Mean age	50–55 years old
Headache characteristics	Thunderclap headache[a]
	Pain is often occipital
Associated features	Seizure
	Nausea/vomiting
	Neck stiffness
	Photophobia
	Loss of consciousness
Physical examination	Elevated blood pressure
	Papilledema and retinal hemorrhages
	Cranial nerve palsies (especially third and sixth nerves)
	Focal neurological deficits
	Seizure
	Decreased level of consciousness

[a] Thunderclap headache defined as acute headache that reaches peak intensity in ≤5 min

Table 3.7 Work-up for suspected SAH

Test	Finding
Non-contrast CT	CT may be negative in 5% of patients evaluated 1 day posthead-ache onset [33]. When CT was performed within 12 h of SAH, one study showed CT failed to detect the SAH for 1.7% of patients [34].
Lumbar puncture (LP)	LP may not detect blood during the first 12 h postbleed; however, CT is most sensitive during this time [39, 40].
Computed tomography angiography (CTA)[a]	Negative noncontrast CT plus CTA excludes SAH with a >99% probability [35].

[a] CTA may be considered as a follow-up test after a negative noncontrast CT in patients for whom a spinal tap cannot be completed or patients without significant risk factors for SAH [35]

Table 3.8 Features suggesting SAH (based on [17])

Series 1	Series 2	Series 3
• Is the patient >40 years old?	• Did the patient arrive by ambulance?	• Did the patient arrive by ambulance?
• Does the patient have neck pain or stiffness?	• Is the patient >45 years old?	• Is the systolic blood pressure >160 mmHg?
• Was there a witnessed loss of consciousness?	• Did the patient vomit at least once?	• Does the patient have neck pain or stiffness?
• Did symptoms begin with exertion?	• Is the diastolic blood pressure >100 mmHg?	• Is the patient between ages 44 and 55?

Answer each series of questions. If one or more of the questions is answered "yes," additional testing for SAH is warranted. If all questions are answered with "no," move to the next series of questions. Make sure all series have been answered "no" before considering the patient to be at low risk for SAH

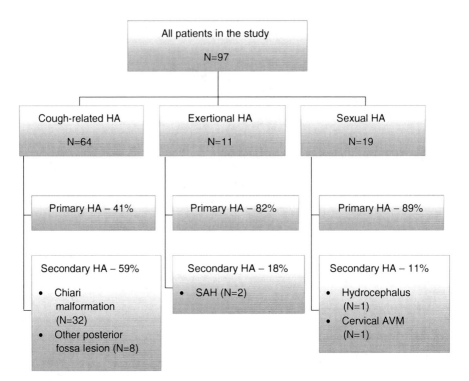

Fig. 3.4 Outcome of 97 patients presenting for headache occurring with cough, exercise, or sexual activity (based on [18]). *AVM* arteriovenous malformation, *HA* headache, *SAH* subarachnoid hemorrhage

diagnosed with a primary headache disorder (54.6%), with a secondary headache occurring in the remainder (45.4%). See Fig. 3.4. Clinical features helped identify patients with primary headache disorders (Table 3.9).

> **Pearl for the practitioner:**
> Among patients with secondary causes for cough-related headache, patients were often younger [mean age at onset = 44 years old] and pain was usually occipital and often lasting <1 min. Patients also often endorsed posterior fossa neurological symptoms, including dizziness, vertigo, facial and upper extremity numbness, and syncope (based on [18]).

Patients presenting with cough, exertional, or sexual headache require imaging of the brain and cerebral vasculature (e.g., magnetic resonance imaging [MRI] and angiography [MRA]) before a primary headache diagnosis can be assigned.

Table 3.9 Characteristics of cough, exertional, and sexual activity associated with primary headache disorder (based on [18])

Cough HA	Exertional HA	Sexual HA
• Not occipital	• Usually bilateral	• Usually bilateral
• No well-defined quality	• Usually pulsating pain	• Usually pulsating pain
• Lasts seconds	• Pain lasts 1 h to 4 days	• Pain lasts 1 min to 4 days
• Always precipitated by cough	• Precipitated by prolonged physical exercise	
• Older patients		
• No associated neurological symptoms		

Fever and Headache

Headache may accompany a wide range of febrile illnesses, including both viral and bacterial infections of structures of the head and neck. Patients with headache caused by infection will typically have signs relating to underlying infectious illness. As noted in Chap. 2, patients often incorrectly attribute migraines to sinus pathology, due to the frequent occurrence of minor autonomic symptoms with migraine. Lack of other signs of infection, such as fever, however, help to identify if infection is likely to be an important contributing or causative factor.

Meningitis

Meningitis is characteristically associated with fever, neck stiffness, and change in mental status (Table 3.10 and Box 3.5). Risk factors are shown in Box 3.6. In a survey of 259 patients with community-acquired bacterial meningitis, only two in three patients had all three of these features (fever, neck stiffness, and change in mental status), while every patient had at least one feature (97% had fever, 88% neck stiffness, 78% had an altered mental status) [19]. In addition, focal seizures or focal neurological findings were identified in 29% of patients on presentation or during the first 24 hours. Typical imaging and pathology findings are shown in Fig. 3.5.

> ***Pearl for the practitioner:***
> In addition to headache, almost all patients with meningitis will also have fever, neck stiffness, or change in mental status. Focal neurological deficits or seizures occur in about one in three patients with meningitis.

Table 3.10 Typical meningitis characteristics

Category	Description
Headache characteristics	Pain worsens with movement or being jostled
Associated features	Pain with moving the eyes
	Nausea/vomiting
	Focal neurological signs
	Rash
Physical examination	Fever
	Neck stiffness
	Altered mental status
	Pain aggravation with jolt test (see Box 3.5)

Box 3.5 Jolt Accentuation Test for Meningitis [37, 38]

- Patient is asked to rotate head horizontally 2–3 times per second
- A positive test occurs when maneuver aggravates a patient's headache
- Sensitivity is 97%; specificity is 60%
- Patients with fever, headache, and positive jolt accentuation should undergo spinal fluid testing, even when neck stiffness and/or altered mental status are absent

Box 3.6 Risk Factors for Meningitis

- Living in groups (e.g., college students or military recruits)
- Trauma or recent neurosurgery
- Other infection (e.g., facial cellulitis, sinusitis, otitis, pneumonia)
- Immune system compromise
- Diabetes
- Alcoholism

A recent literature review of acute meningitis showed that clinical history alone is generally inadequate to confirm a diagnosis of meningitis. Physical examination, however, is usually helpful although the study reported above and others reviewed in this report similarly showed that most patients will typically not have the full triad of meningitis signs on examination. The diagnosis, however, could be ruled out in patients failing to have any of the three signs.

Pearl for the practitioner:
While many patients will not have all three of the hallmark triad signs for meningitis (fever, neck stiffness, and altered mental status), they should have at least one to consider this diagnosis.

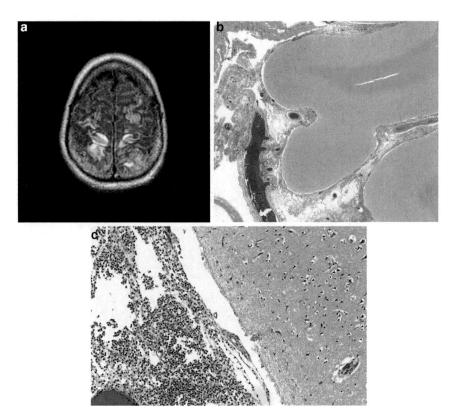

Fig. 3.5 Meningitis (images courtesy of Clayton A. Wiley, MD, PhD). (**a**) Magnetic resonance imaging, horizontal section. This image of the top of the head demonstrates bright signal along the surface of the brain conforming to the gyri and sulci. This signal is consistent with intense inflammation within the meninges along the surface of the brain. (**b**) Pathology of meningeal sample, low power. This low-power image is of a hematoxylin (*blue*) and eosin (*red*) stained section from the surface of the brain of a patient with acute meningitis. On the left side, a large vessel is filled with red bloods cells and surrounded by a dense collection of inflammatory cells. The inflammation is limited to the surface of the brain and does not penetrate into the tissue. (**c**) Pathology of meningeal sample, high power. This high-power image is of a hematoxylin (*blue*) and eosin (*red*) stained section from the surface of the brain of a patient with acute meningitis. The *left side* shows a dense collection of inflammatory cells forming a pool of pus on the surface of the brain. The brain tissue adjacent to the inflammatory cells is bathed in potent cytokines from the inflammatory cells that will compromise its function

Bacterial meningitis can be a rapidly progressive, fulminant, and even fatal infection (Fig. 3.6). The European Federation of Neurological Societies (EFNS) published a flow chart detailing the emergency management of patients with suspected bacterial meningitis that provides a useful assessment algorithm (Fig. 3.7) [20]. Empirical antibiotic treatment for suspected acute bacterial meningitis is given in Box 3.7.

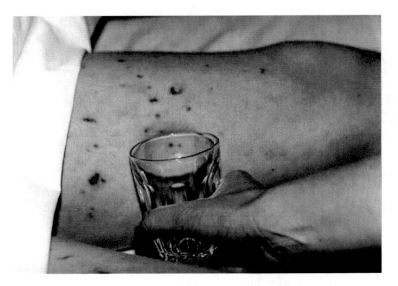

Fig. 3.6 A nonblanching, petechial rash is characteristic of meningococcal meningitis. This rash often begins as a diffuse, erythematous, maculopapular rash that evolves into petechiae and purpura on the trunk and lower extremities. As seen in the photo, this rash does not fade under pressure (photo courtesy of The Meningitis Trust)

Vascular Disease

Headache may occur in patients presenting with ischemic or hemorrhagic stroke, cerebral venous or dural sinus thrombosis. Stroke risk is increased in patients with migraine [21]. Migraineurs have been shown to have significantly increased risk for cardiovascular disease, as well as a variety of cardiovascular risk factors, including diabetes, hypertension, and hypercholesterolemia [22]. After controlling for potentially confounding factors, including cardiovascular risk factors, migraine with or without aura is still linked to increased risk for cardiovascular disease (Fig. 3.8).

Cerebral Venous Thrombosis

Cerebral venous thrombosis is a rare cause of stroke, typically affecting adults <50 years old. Patients with cerebral venous thrombosis may present with stroke, headache, or cranial nerve palsies. Headache is usually diffuse and progressive over days to weeks [23]. Seizures are also common, affecting about 40% of cases [23]. In general, pain does not lateralize to the side of the thrombus (Table 3.11) [24]. Patients should be screened for the presence of congenital or acquired risk factors (Table 3.12) [25]. Patients with suspected cerebral venous thrombosis should be screened for a hypercoagulable state [23]. Diagnosis is typically made after reviewing imaging studies. Noncontrast CT or MRI testing will characteristically show

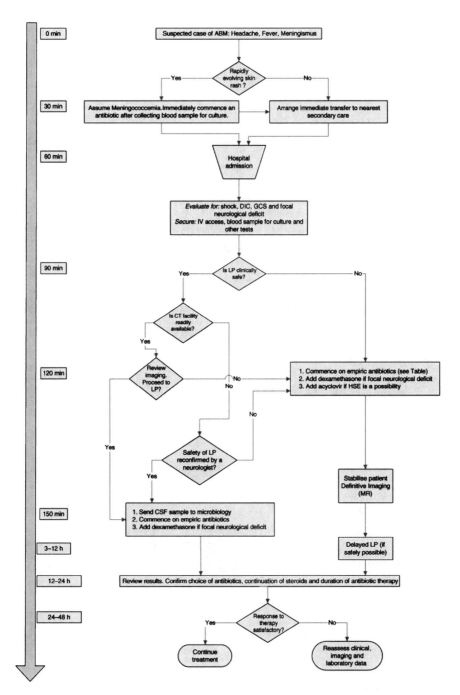

Fig. 3.7 EFNS flow chart for ED management of suspected bacterial meningitis (reprinted with permission from [20]). The arrow on the left shows the time course anticipated for the average evaluation in minutes (min) and hours (h). For the treatment "Table" referred to in the flow chart, please refer to Box 3.7. *ABM* acute bacterial meningitis, *CSF* cerebrospinal fluid, *CT* computed tomography, *DIC* disseminated intravascular coagulation, *GCS* Glasgow Coma Scale, *HSE* herpes simplex encephalitis, *IV* intravenous, *LP* lumbar puncture, *MR* magnetic resonance imaging

Box 3.7 EFNS Recommendations for Empiric Treatment of Suspected Acute Bacterial Meningitis (Based on [20]). *IM* intramuscular, *IV* intravenous

• Ceftriaxone 2 g every 12–24 hours or cefotaxime 2 g every 6–8 hours

  – An alternative therapy would be meropenem 2 g every 8 hours or chloramphenicol 1 g every 6 hours

• If penicillin or cephalosporin-resistant pneumococcus is suspected, use ceftriaxone or cefotaxime plus vancomycin 60 mg/kg every 24 hours (adjusted for creatinine clearance) after loading dose of 15 mg/kg
• Ampicillin/amoxicillin 2 g every 4 hours if *Listeria* is suspected (e.g., elderly and immunosuppressed patients)
• If spinal fluid analysis needs to be delayed/postponed (e.g., signs or symptoms of increased intracranial pressure)

  – Antibiotics should be started after obtaining blood cultures
  – IV or IM benzyl penicillin
  – IV cefotaxime or ceftriaxone

• Patients allergic to beta-lactams may be treated with vancomycin for likely pneumococcal meningitis and chloramphenicol for likely meningococcal meningitis
• Dexamethasone may be an appropriate adjunctive therapy after initial antibiotic dosing

Fig. 3.8 Significantly increased risk for cardiovascular disease among migraineurs, after controlling for gender, age, disability, treatment, and cardiovascular disease risk factors (based on [22]). An odds ratio >1 signifies increased risk

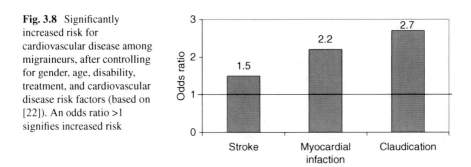

ischemic infarction that does not correspond to an arterial distribution. Evidence of thrombosed veins or clotted blood in the sinuses is usually not seen. Magnetic resonance testing is more sensitive for detecting cerebral venous thrombosis than CT [23]. Diagnosis can be confirmed with CT angiography. Lumbar puncture is generally not necessary; however, clues to possible cerebral venous thrombosis in headache patients in the ED who have had a lumbar puncture include elevations in opening pressure, cell count, and protein, although these abnormalities are not uniformly present [23]. After diagnosis, cerebral venous thrombosis is managed with medical stabilization and consultation with neurology/neurosurgery.

Table 3.11 Typical features
in patients with proven
cerebral venous thrombosis
(based on [24])

Category	Percentage
Pain quality	
Band-like	38
Throbbing	17
Thunderclap	10
Other	36
Pain location	
Unilateral	48
Diffuse	28
Localized	25
Neurological findings	
No abnormalities	32
Papilledema	15
Altered mental status	19
Focal deficit	22

Table 3.12 Risk factors for cerebral venous thrombosis (based on [25] and [23])

Congenital factors	Acquired factors
• Activated protein C resistance and factor V Leiden mutation	• Coagulopathy, including use of oral contraceptives and pregnancy
• Antiphospholipid and anticardiolipin antibodies	• Dehydration (especially in children)
• Elevated prothrombin (e.g., prothrombin G20210A mutation)	• Hematological disorders (e.g., iron deficiency anemia, polycythemia, thrombocythemia, nephrotic syndrome)
• Hyperhomocysteinemia	• Infection of structures of the head or central nervous system
• Protein C, protein S, and antithrombin deficiencies	• Inflammatory disease (e.g., systemic lupus erythematosus, sarcoidosis, and inflammatory bowel disease)
	• Malignancy
	• Mechanical complications from lumbar puncture or epidural blood patch
	• Medications (e.g., androgens, corticosteroids, phytoestrogens, danazol, erythropoietin, vitamin A, lithium, tamoxifen, L-asparaginase, intravenous immunoglobulin, ecstasy)
	• Systemic illness (e.g., Lupus, Behçet disease, inflammatory bowel disease, thyroid disease, sarcoidosis)
	• Trauma or cranial surgery

Increased Intracranial Pressure

Increased intracranial pressure may occur due to mass lesions or idiopathic intracranial hypertension. The presence of papilledema and neurological deficits on examination suggests increased intracranial pressure and often a mass lesion. Patients with marked increased intracranial hypertension may develop temporary blindness typically lasting <1 min called *transient visual obscurations*. Visual obscurations typically occur when patients stand from a sitting position.

Headache in patients with mass lesions is often nonspecific and difficult to distinguish from primary headaches based on headache features alone [26]. The presence of abnormal symptoms or signs (e.g., neurological deficits) help to determine patients with likely intracranial mass lesions who will require additional testing.

Idiopathic Intracranial Hypertension

Idiopathic intracranial hypertension was previously referred to as *pseudotumor cerebri* or *benign intracranial hypertension*. Idiopathic intracranial hypertension refers to markedly increased intracranial pressure unrelated to inflammatory or structural pathology. Surveys of patients with idiopathic intracranial hypertension in both Europe and the USA show remarkably similar patient demographics, with most patients being obese women of reproductive age (Table 3.13) [27, 28]. Typical symptoms of presentation are shown in Table 3.14 and Fig. 3.9. A recent survey of

Table 3.13 Typical characteristics of idiopathic intracranial hypertension (based on [28] and [27])

Category	Description
Mean age	34 years old
Female gender	90–92%
Comorbid obesity	88–100%
Other comorbid conditions	Addison's disease
	Dural sinus thrombosis
	Hyperparathyroidism
	Hypervitaminosis A
	Menarche
	Phenothiazine treatment
	Polycystic ovarian syndrome
	Pregnancy
	Recent weight gain
	Steroid treatment or withdrawal
	Tetracycline treatment
Headache characteristics	Diffuse, constant head pain
	Headache aggravated by coughing, straining, Valsalva, or rising from sitting (rising from sitting may be accompanied by transient visual obscurations)
Physical examination	Papilledema
	Sixth nerve palsy
	Markedly increased pressure reading on lumbar puncture performed in the lateral decubitus position (Table 3.15) with normal spinal fluid chemistry and cell count
	Symptomatic relief after reduction in intracranial pressure through spinal fluid drainage

Table 3.14 Presenting symptoms in patients with idiopathic intracranial hypertension (based on [36])

Presenting symptom	Percentage of patients
Headache	76
Transient visual obscurations	48
Vision loss	48
Nausea/vomiting	30
Diplopia	8

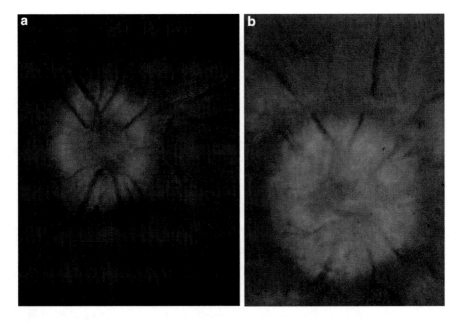

Fig. 3.9 Papilledema (photos courtesy of Rock Heyman, MD). (**a**) Papilledema with loss of clear vascular markings and blurring of the optic disc. (**b**) Severe papilledema in patient with idiopathic intracranial hypertension showing obliteration of vascular markings

159 women diagnosed with idiopathic intracranial hypertension reported a mean weight during the year before diagnosis of 92 kg, with an average weight gain of 5 kg over the year before diagnosis [29]. Visual field abnormalities were identified at diagnosis in 84% of these patients, highlighting the important effect this condition has on vision. Opening cerebrospinal fluid pressure is used to confirm intracranial hypertension, with indicative pressures varying by age (Table 3.15) [30]. Lumbar puncture may be more easily accomplished in obese patients in the leaning forward position; however, accurate interpretation of opening pressure is limited in this position. If a diagnostic tap cannot be achieved in the lateral decubitus position, it may be worthwhile to seek neurology consultation to assist with lumbar puncture and diagnosis confirmation. Treatment focuses on achieving and maintaining more normal pressures (Box 3.8).

Table 3.15 Elevated lumbar pressures suggesting idiopathic intracranial hypertension vary by age (based on [30])

Age	Abnormal pressure suggesting idiopathic intracranial hypertension (mmH$_2$O)
Children <8 years old	>180
Children ≥8 years old	>250
Adults	>250

Box 3.8 Treatment Recommendations for Idiopathic Intracranial Hypertension

- ED treatment
  - Spinal fluid drainage to reduce intracranial pressure
  - Referral to neurology and ophthalmology
- Chronic management focuses on reducing pressures to prevent permanent visual loss
  - Correction of any underlying predisposing condition(s)
  - Weight loss in overweight/obese patients
  - Acetazolamide
  - Repeated lumbar puncture
  - Lumboperitoneal or ventriculoperitoneal shunting in select patients
  - Optic nerve sheath fenestration in select patients

Giant Cell or Temporal Arteritis

Giant cell arteritis (also called temporal arteritis) is an inflammatory condition that typically occurs at or after age 50, with most affected individuals >70 years old [31]. Women are affected over twice as often as men [32]. Giant cell arteritis should be considered in all patients ≥50 years old presenting to the ED for headache. Giant cell arteritis is described in detail in Chap. 7.

Other Secondary Headaches

Other secondary headaches to consider, especially in adults >50 years old, include primary and metastatic malignancies, acute glaucoma, CO poisoning, and anginal equivalents involving head and neck pain.

Table 3.16 At-a-glance clues to identify common secondary headaches

Secondary headache	Demographics and precipitants	Symptoms	Signs
Acute angle-closure glaucoma	Asians and Eskimos at higher risk Females Seniors	Severe eye pain Nausea Tearing Blurred vision; seeing "halos"	Red eye
Carbon monoxide poisoning	Other members in household are similarly affected. More common during winter months in poorly ventilated areas	Headache Dizziness Flu-like symptoms Abdominal pain Fatigue Confusion	Flushing Mental status changes
Cervicocranial arterial dissection	Head or neck trauma, neck hyperextension, spinal manipulation	Pain Stroke-syndrome	Deficits based on vascular distribution affected
Cerebral venous/sinus thrombosis	Coagulopathy Pregnancy Dehydration Cranial infection	Band-like headache Often unilateral pain	Focal deficits Mental status changes Papilledema
Giant cell arteritis	Adult ≥50 years old	Head pain and tenderness Change in vision Jaw pain with chewing	Prominent and tender temple vessels Fever Elevated ESR or CRP
Idiopathic intracranial hypertension	Obesity Female	Transient blindness abruptly with standing	Marked papilledema Sixth nerve palsy
Preeclampsia	Pregnancy, postpartum	Hand or face swelling Dizziness Right upper abdominal/rib pain Vision changes	Hypertension Proteinuria
Subarachnoid hemorrhage	Adult 50–55 years old	Thunderclap headache Occipital pain Neck stiffness Photophobia	Seizure Hypertension Decreased level of consciousness Focal neurological deficits

CRP C-reactive protein, *ESR* erythrocyte sedimentation rate

Malignancy

Older adults with additional systemic symptoms, such as weight loss, poor appetite, fever, and unexplained masses or bleeding should be investigated for possible cancer. Headaches can occur due to primary or metastatic malignancies involving the brain.

Acute Angle-Closure Glaucoma

Acute angle-closure glaucoma should be suspected when patients, particularly older adults, present complaining of decreased vision, headaches, seeing "halos" around lights, severe eye pain, and/or nausea and vomiting. Physical findings can include conjunctival redness, corneal edema, and sluggish reaction of pupils to light. Patients with suspected acute glaucoma should be referred immediately to an ophthalmologist.

Carbon Monoxide (CO) Poisoning

CO poisoning should be considered for patients presenting with headaches, malaise, mental status changes, confusion, seizures, nausea, and/or dizziness, particularly during winter months in colder climates when poorly functioning heating systems, kerosene heaters, charcoal grills, camping stoves, and/or gas powered electrical generators and cars may be used in poorly ventilated areas. Diagnosis is made based on history and CO oximetry or a breath analyzer. Carboxyhemoglobin can also be measured directly. Importantly, pulse oximetry should NOT be relied upon to measure oxygen in suspected CO poisoning, as pulse oximetry cannot distinguish between carboxyhemoglobin and oxyhemoglobin and thus may give false normal results for a severely anoxic patient. ECG can show ischemic changes. Treatment is 100% oxygen.

Anginal Equivalent Presenting as Headache

Another secondary headache not to be missed in adults is an anginal equivalent. If the headache is related to exertion and is relieved with rest, particularly in a person with documented coronary artery disease (CAD) history or significant CAD risk factors, anginal equivalent should be considered.

Summary

- Patients with mild traumatic brain injury need to receive instructions on the need for mental and physical rest, as well as for specific recommendations about resuming sports activities.
- Cervicocranial artery dissection can occur after seemingly minor neck trauma. Dissection typically results in headache with symptoms suggesting ischemic stroke or SAH.
- Benign headache is the most common diagnosis in patients with thunderclap headache. Because clinical features poorly distinguish between benign and serious thunderclap headache (e.g., SAH), all patients presenting with their first episode of thunderclap headache require a brain CT and spinal fluid testing, when CT testing is negative.

- Although patients with meningitis often fail to have the full triad of fever, neck stiffness, and altered mental status, they should have at least one of these signs.
- Idiopathic intracranial hypertension refers to markedly increased intracranial pressure unrelated to inflammatory or structural pathology that typically occurs in obese females in their younger adult years. This is diagnosed in patients with papilledema, a normal brain imaging study, and markedly elevated opening pressure on lumbar puncture performed in the lateral decubitus position.
- All older adults presenting to the ED with a new headache should be evaluated for possible giant cell arteritis and primary/metastatic malignancy.

References

1. Ruff RM, Iverson GL, Barth JT, et al. Recommendations for diagnosing a mild traumatic brain injury: a National Academy of Neuropsychology Education paper. Arch Clin Neuropsychol. 2009;24:3–10.
2. Jagoda AS, Bazarian JJ, Bruns JJ, et al. Clinical Policy: Neuroimaging and decisionmaking in adult mild traumatic brain injury in the acute setting. Ann Emerg Med. 2008;52:714–48.
3. McCrory P, Meeuwisse W, Johnston K, et al. Consensus statement on concussion in sport: the 3rd International Conference on Concussion in Sport held in Zurich, November 2008. Br J Sports Med. 2009;43 Suppl 1:i76–84.
4. Randolph C. Baseline neuropsychological testing in managing sport-related concussion: does it modify risk? Curr Sports Med Rep. 2011;10:21–6.
5. Covassin T, Elbin RJ, Stiller-Ostrowski JL, Kontos AP. Immediate post-concussion assessment and cognitive testing (ImPACT) practices of sports medicine professional. J Athl Train. 2009;44:639–44.
6. Jensen MB, Chacon MR, Aleu A. Cervicocerebral arterial dissection. Neurologist. 2008;14:5–6.
7. Caso V, Paciaroni M, Bogousslavsky J. Environmental factors and cervical artery dissection. Front Neurol Neurosci. 2005;20:44–53.
8. Dharmasaronja P, Dharmasaroja P. Sports-related internal carotid artery dissection. Pathogenesis and therapeutic point of view. Neurologist. 2008;14:307–11.
9. Haneline M, Triano J. Cervical artery dissection. A comparison of highly dynamic mechanisms: manipulation versus motor vehicle collision. J Manipulative Physiol Ther. 2005;28:57–63.
10. Schievink WI. Spontaneous dissection of the carotid and vertebral arteries. N Engl J Med. 2001;344:898–906.
11. Shah Q, Messé SR. Cervicocranial arterial dissection. Curr Treat Options Neurol. 2007;9:55–62.
12. Huang Y, Chen Y, Wang Y, et al. Cervicocranial arterial dissection: experience of 73 patients in a single center. Surg Neurol. 2009;72 Suppl 2:S20–7.
13. Shah Q, Messé SR. Cervicocranial arterial dissection. Curr Treat Option Neurol. 2007;9:55–62.
14. Linn FH, Rinkel GE, Algra A, van Gijn J. Headache characteristics in subarachnoid haemorrhage and benign thunderclap headache. J Neurol Neurosurg Psychiatry. 1998;65:791–3.
15. Landtblom AM, Fridriksson S, Boivie J, et al. Sudden onset headache: a prospective study of features, incidence and causes. Cephalalgia. 2002;22:354–60.
16. Perry JJ, Stiell IG, Wells GA, et al. Attitudes and judgment of emergency physicians in the management of patients with acute headache. Acad Emerg Med. 2005;12:33–7.
17. Perry JJ, Stiell IG, Sivilotti ML, et al. High risk clinical characteristics for subarachnoid haemorrhage in patients with acute headache: prospective cohort study. BMJ. 2010;341:c5204.

18. Pascual J, González-Mandly A, Martín R, Oterino A. Headaches precipitated by cough, prolonged exercise or sexual activity: a prospective etiological and clinical study. J Headache Pain. 2008;9:259–66.
19. Durand ML, Calderwood SB, Weber DJ, et al. Acute bacterial meningitis in adults. A review of 493 episodes. N Engl J Med. 1993;328:21–8.
20. Chaudhuri A, Martin PM, Kennedy GE, et al. EFNS guideline on the management of community acquired bacterial meningitis: report of an EFNS Task Force on acute bacterial meningitis in older children and adults. Eur J Neurol. 2008;15:649–59.
21. Kurth T. The association of migraine with ischemic stroke. Curr Neurol Neurosci Rep. 2010;10:133–9.
22. Bigal ME, Kurth T, Santanello N, et al. Migraine and cardiovascular disease: a population-based study. Neurology. 2010;74:628–35.
23. Saposnik G, Barinagarrementeria F, Brown RD, et al. Diagnosis and management of cerebral venous thrombosis. A statement for healthcare professionals from the American Heart Association/American Stroke Association. Stroke. 2011;42:1158–92.
24. Wasay M, Kojan S, Dai AI, Bobustuc G, Sheikh Z. Headache in cerebral venous thrombosis: incidence, pattern and location in 200 consecutive patients. J Headache Pain. 2010;11:137–9.
25. McBane RD, Tafur A, Wysokinski WE. Acquired and congenital risk factors associated with cerebral venous sinus thrombosis. Thromb Res. 2010;126:81–7.
26. Valentinis L, Tuniz F, Valent F, et al. Headache attributed to intracranial tumours: a prospective study. Cephalalgia. 2010;30:389–98.
27. Asensio-Sánchez VM, Merino-Angulo J, Martínez-Calvo S, Calvo MJ, Rodríguez R. Epidemiology of pseudotumor cerebri. Arch Soc Esp Oftalmol. 2007;82:219–21.
28. Galvin JA, Van Stavern GP. Clinical characterization of idiopathic intracranial hypertension at the Detroit Medical Center. J Neurol Sci. 2004;223:157–60.
29. Baldwin MK, Lobb B, Tanne E, Egan R. Weight and visual field deficits in women with idiopathic intracranial hypertension. J Womens Health (Larchmt). 2010;19:1893–8.
30. Rangwala LM, Liu GT. Pediatric idiopathic intracranial hypertension. Surv Ophthalmol. 2007;52:597–617.
31. González-Gay MA, Garcia-Porrua C, Rivas MJ, Rodriguez-Ledo P, Llorca J. Epidemiology of biopsy proven giant cell arteritis in northwestern Spain: trend over an 18 year period. Ann Rheum Dis. 2001;60:367–71.
32. Salvarani C, Corwson CS, O'Fallon M, Hunder GG, Gabriel SE. Reappraisal of the epidemiology of giant cell arteritis in Olmsted County, Minnesota, over a fifty-year period. Arthritis Rheum. 2004;51:264–8.
33. Adams Jr HP, Kassell NF, Torner JC, Sahs AL. CT and clinical correlations in recent aneurysmal subarachnoid hemorrhage: a preliminary report of the Cooperative Aneurysm Study. Neurology. 1983;33:981–8.
34. van der Wee N, Rinkel GE, Hasan D, van Gijn J. Detection of subarachnoid haemorrhage on early CT: is lumbar puncture still needed after a negative scan? J Neurol Neurosurg Psychiatry. 1995;58:357–9.
35. McCormack RF, Hutson A. Can computed tomography angiography of the brain replace lumbar puncture in the evaluation of acute-onset headache after a negative noncontrast cranial computed tomography scan. Acad Emerg Med. 2010;17:444–51.
36. Ambika S, Arjundas D, Noronha V, Anshuman. Clinical profile, evaluation, management and visual outcome of idiopathic intracranial hypertension in a neuro-ophthalmology clinic of a tertiary referral ophthalmic center in India. Ann Indian Acad Neurol. 2010;13(1):37–41.
37. Uchihara T, Tsukagoshi H. Jolt accentuation of headache: the most sensitive sign of CSF pleocytosis. Headache. 1991;31:167–71.
38. Fitch MT, van de Beek D. Emergency diagnosis and treatment of adult meningitis. Lancet Infect Dis. 2007;7:191–200.
39. Schull MJ. Diagnostic dilemmas and subarachnoid hemorrhage subtleties: What to do when the evidence gives you a headache. CJEM. 2002;4:106–7.
40. Liebenberg WA, Worth R, Firth GB, Olney J, Norris JS. Aneurysmal subarachnoid haemorrhage: guidance in making the correct diagnosis. Postgrad Med J 2005;81:470–3.

Chapter 4
General Treatment Strategies

Key chapter points

- Initial treatment for patients with non-traumatic, primary headache includes rehydration and aggressive treatment of nausea.
- Patients with severe headache pain may need treatment with headache-specific therapies (i.e., triptans or dihydroergotamine) or non-opioid analgesics (i.e., ketorolac).
- Additional options include intravenous magnesium, intravenous valproate, trigger point injections, and occipital nerve blocks.
- Steroids offer minimal benefit, although intravenous dexamethasone may help patients with disabling primary headache lasting over 3 days.
- Opioids should be reserved for rescue therapy in the ED and not routinely provided as take-home medication.

Keywords Anti-emetic • Hydration • Injection • Occipital nerve block • Trigger point

After ruling out important causes of secondary headache, the emergency department (ED) management of the headache patient focuses on symptomatic treatment. General principles for ED treatment of migraine include:

- Treating dehydration;
- Treating nausea aggressively;
- Using nonmedication pain-reducing therapies;
- Using a rational polypharmacy approach to maximize treatment efficacy;
- Avoiding the routine use of opioid medications for pain and not providing opioid medications as take-home medications;
- Considering trigger point injections or occipital nerve blocks for patients with recalcitrant headaches.

D.A. Marcus and P.A. Bain, *Practical Assessment and Treatment of the Patient with Headaches in the Emergency Department and Urgent Care Clinic*, DOI 10.1007/978-1-4614-0002-8_4, © Springer Science+Business Media, LLC 2011

Throughout this chapter, studies will be presented that may use different endpoints to describe symptomatic improvement. *Pain relief* is defined as a reduction in pain severity to mild or no pain, while a *pain-free* response describes complete resolution of pain. Furthermore, a reduction in headache pain by at least 50% is generally considered to represent a *clinically meaningful* improvement.

Treating Dehydration

Associated nausea and vomiting often accompany severe migraine. Dehydration may be a headache trigger [1] or a consequence of prolonged migraine-related nausea and vomiting. Dehydration is linked to increased headache activity [2, 3], while increasing water intake decreases headache severity and frequency [4]. Anecdotally, intravenous rehydration is an important component of ED headache treatment. Typically, administration of intravenous normal saline at 200 mL/h can help reverse dehydration.

> *Pearl for the practitioner:*
> Many patients presenting to the ED with acute headache are dehydrated, even when nausea and vomiting are not major complaints. Intravenous rehydration can help reduce symptoms.

> **Box 4.1** Obtaining Intravenous Access for Treating Dehydration and Administering Medications
>
> Intravenous (IV) access is often necessary in the ED headache patient for rehydration and medication administration. Gastric stasis during migraine attacks can reduce the efficacy of oral therapies [70]. The following tips can help secure intravenous access in dehydrated patients:
>
> - Assess the potential veins for cannulation with the tourniquet in place
> - Have the patient open and close their fist numerous times
> - Select high-yield sites for access in the following order: forearm, medial cubital, dorsum of the foot, saphenous veins in the lower extremity (lower limb veins should generally be used as a last resort)
> - Take advantage of dependency: dangle the arm for 1–2 min below the level of the heart
> - Use a blood pressure cuff at a low setting ~60 mmHg about 3 finger breadths above the vein
> - Use palpation in addition to visualizing veins
> - Prevent vein rolling by applying pressure by holding traction below the IV insertion site

(continued)

> **Box 4.1** (continued)
>
> - Use EMLA cream to reduce discomfort, applying as long before IV insertion as possible
> - Dilate veins with warmth. Try a warming blanket, warm moist towels, or fill a disposable glove with warm water and tape to extremity for a period of time (many institutions frown on using microwave to heat the towels for fear that towels will become too hot)
> - Learn ultrasound-guided technique for really difficult cases
> - Hand-held vein transilluminator devices can be helpful (e.g., Veinlite [http://www.veinlite.com/])
>
> When venous access cannot be achieved, select headache treatments that may be administered intramuscularly or subcutaneously, such as ondansetron, prochlorperazine, ketorolac, and sumatriptan.

Treating Nausea Aggressively

Antinausea medications can help relieve both nausea and pain associated with severe migraine headaches in the ED (Table 4.1). There are two main classes of antinausea drugs: anti-emetics and anti-emetics with additional pain relieving properties.

Table 4.1 Anti-emetics for migraine

Anti-emetic	Typical adult dosing
First-line parenteral agents	
Metoclopramide	10 mg IV over several minutes or IM
Prochlorperazine	10 mg IV over 2–5 min
Trimethobenzamide	200 mg IM
First-line rectal suppositories	
Chlorpromazine	50–100 mg suppository
Promethazine	25 mg suppository
Other options	
Chlorpromazine	25 mg IV
Droperidol[a]	2.5 mg IM or IV
Haloperidol	5 mg IM or IV
Olanzapine	2.5–5 mg orally
Quetiapine	50–100 mg orally

Extrapyramidal side effects can be reduced by pre-treating or concomitantly treating intravenously or intramuscularly with 25 mg diphenhydramine or 1 mg benztropine. Administering these drugs slowly may help reduce the risk for developing akathisia

IM intramuscular injection, *IV* intravenous dosing

[a]Due to black box warning, pretreatment electrocardiogram is needed to ensure QT_c <450 ms. Droperidol should also be avoided in patients with low potassium or magnesium levels

Ondansetron (Zofran) is a very effective, well-tolerated anti-emetic that is often an excellent first choice for nausea because of its tolerability. Medications such as metoclopramide (Reglan) and phenothiazines prochlorperazine (Compazine) and promethazine (Phenergan) additionally reduce headache pain and nausea because of their antidopaminergic activity. Akathisia, a feeling of inner restlessness, is a common side effect with dopaminergic anti-emetics that patients should be directly asked about. Nearly two of every three ED practitioners report using diphenhydramine (Benadryl) as adjunctive therapy when using dopaminergic anti-emetics to minimize akathisia [5].

Although patients presenting to the ED for migraine typically focus on pain symptoms, a systematic review and meta-analysis comparing outcome in studies treating migraine patients with parenteral phenothiazines (chlorpromazine [Thorazine] or prochlorperazine) vs. other parenteral agents (including metoclopramide, ketorolac [Toradol], sumatriptan [Imitrex], meperidine [Demerol], or valproate [Depacon]) showed increased likelihood of successful treatment with phenothiazines (odds ratio = 2.04, 95% confidence interval [CI] 1.25–3.31) [6]. Achieving a pain-free response was similar between phenothiazines and other treatments. Phenothiazines were likewise better than metoclopramide (OR 2.25, 95% CI 1.29–3.92) for overall success, although complete pain freedom was again similar.

> **Pearl for the practitioner:**
> Nausea should be treated aggressively in patients presenting with acute headache to the ED. Ondansetron is a well-tolerated medication that treats only the nausea. Phenothiazines and metoclopramide effectively treat nausea as well as pain.

A randomized study showed similar efficacy with intravenous treatment of acute migraine with 10 mg prochlorperazine or 20 mg metoclopramide, both drugs administered in conjunction with 25 mg of intravenous diphenhydramine [7]. Pain relief was achieved by about half of treated patients, with nausea relief in nearly every patient (Fig. 4.1). Other studies have shown that intramuscular droperidol (Inapsine) is more effective in relieving headache-related pain than prochlorperazine [8] and as effective as meperidine (Demerol) [9].

While droperidol is an excellent medication for nausea and headache pain, it has been associated with cases of QT prolongation and ventricular arrhythmias, with a Food and Drug Administration (FDA) black box warning issued. Droperidol use should, therefore, be limited with an electrocardiogram obtained prior to administration with continuous QT monitoring while in the ED. QT prolongation has also been reported with phenothiazines and ondansetron [10–12]. Furthermore, prochlorperazine

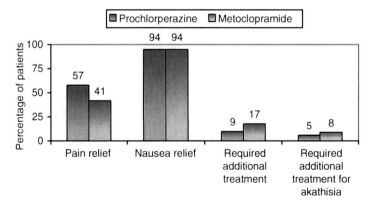

Fig. 4.1 ED treatment with intravenous prochlorperazine 10 mg vs. metoclopramide 20 mg (based on [7]). Endpoints were measured 2 h after initial treatment. Nausea relief was measured in the 91% of patients who were nauseated at baseline. None of the numeric differences were significant

Pearl for the practitioner:
Akathisia and other extrapyramidal side effects that may occur can be reduced by

- Giving phenothiazines or metoclopramide slowly over 30–60 min
- Pretreating with diphenhydramine

is often preferred over chlorpromazine, due to marked orthostasis that may occur with chlorpromazine. Giving a fluid bolus before administering chlorpromazine can reduce hypotension. Antipsychotics, including better tolerated atypical antipsychotics (e.g., olanzapine and quetiapine), may also be used for migraine treatment when needed, although usually as less preferred therapy due to side effects [13].

Anti-emetics Are More Effective for ED Headache Than Analgesics

Studies suggest that anti-emetic therapies, such as metoclopramide or phenothiazines, are more effective than treatment with analgesics. A retrospective chart review showed superior pain relief in patients treated with metoclopramide compared with hydromorphone (Dilaudid; Fig. 4.2) [14]. In all cases, metoclopramide was administered intravenously, while hydromorphone was intravenous for 94% and

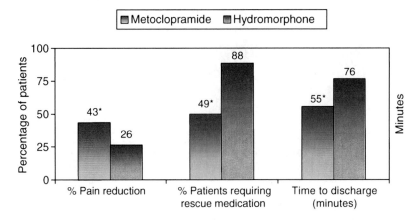

Fig. 4.2 ED treatment with anti-emetic vs. opioid (based on [14]). All differences were significant (*$P < 0.01$) and favored metoclopramide

intramuscular for 6% of patients. Another study similarly reported superior efficacy with metoclopramide compared with pethidine (meperidine) [15].

Anti-emetics Are At Least as Effective as Triptans for ED Migraine

Improvement in pain for ED migraine treatment has been shown to be at least as good with anti-emetics as triptan treatment. For example, high-dose metoclopramide and the combination of trimethobenzamide (Tigan) plus diphenhydramine were each as effective as subcutaneous sumatriptan in randomized, double-blind clinical trials (Fig. 4.3) [16, 17]. Another randomized, double-blind study showed similar good benefits in patients treated with 500 mL saline and then randomized to either 10 mg prochlorperazine plus 12.5 mg diphenhydramine intravenously or 6 mg sumatriptan subcutaneously for acute migraine in the ED [18]. Pain was reduced by 96% with prochlorperazine and 70% with sumatriptan. Although only 61% of treated patients could be contacted for follow-up, headache had returned within 72 h for 43% treated with prochlorperazine and 63% with sumatriptan.

> **Pearl for the practitioner:**
> Metoclopramide and phenothiazines are at least as effective as subcutaneous sumatriptan and more effective than opioid analgesics for the treatment of ED migraine.

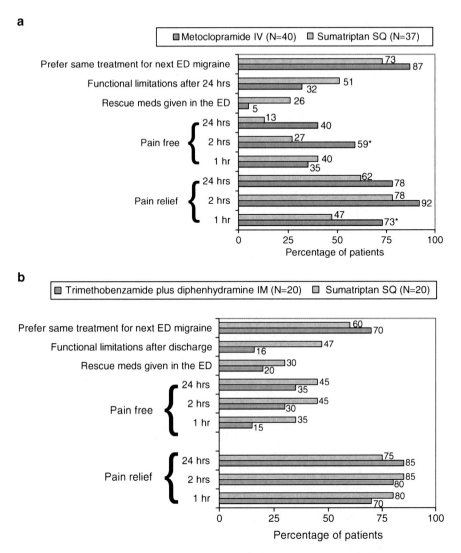

Fig. 4.3 ED treatment with anti-emetic vs. sumatriptan. For both studies, pain relief describes a reduction of pain severity to mild or none, while pain free describes reduction of pain severity to none. (**a**) Intravenous (IV) metoclopramide 20 mg dosed up to four times vs. subcutaneous (SQ) sumatriptan 6 mg (based on [16]). *Numerical differences favoring metoclopramide over sumatriptan were statistically significant at two time points ($P<0.05$). (**b**) Intramuscular (IM) trimethobenzamide 200 mg plus diphenhydramine 25 mg vs. subcutaneous (SQ) sumatriptan 6 mg (based on [17]). None of these numerical differences was significant

Include Nondrug Treatments

Routinely incorporating simple nondrug treatments can improve patient comfort and treatment satisfaction [19]. Headache-provoking external stimulation can be decreased by:

- Promptly taking headache patients to private rooms with dimmed lighting;
- Offering ice packs for the patient to put on the forehead or neck;
- Having family members or friends perform neck massage if cutaneous allodynia is not present;
- Educating the ED staff to offer patient instruction in relaxation exercises (Box 4.2) and gentle cervical range of motion exercises (Box 4.3);
- Presenting information in a positive rather than negative or neutral manner. For example, replace statements like, "I hope that this will help" or "This might work" with more positive wording like, "This medication is often very effective" or "Many people really respond well to this treatment."

Box 4.2 Relaxation Techniques

- Instruct the patient to sit quietly without crossing arms or legs
- Ask the patient to close her eyes
- Give these instructions for cue-controlled relaxation, which combines deep breathing and repetition of the word "relax"
  - Take a slow, deep, abdominal breath
  - Place your hand over your stomach while you breath slowly and deeply
  - Make sure you feel your stomach moving in and out with each breath
  - After breathing in, hold your breath for 5–10 s, then breath out, slowly repeating the word "relax"
  - Repeat this for 10–15 min
- Give these instructions for progressive muscle relaxation, which has the patient alternatively contract and relax muscles
  - Tighten the muscles in your feet
  - Focus on how the muscles feel when tensed
  - Hold the tension for 10–15 s
  - Release the tension and feel the muscles relax
  - Focus on how the muscle feels once relaxed
  - Now tighten the muscles in your legs. Hold for 10–15 s and then relax
  - Repeat this process with muscles in your abdomen, then your arms, then your shoulders, then your neck, then your jaw, then your eyes, and finally your forehead
  - Focus on how the muscles in your body feel when they are no longer tensed

Box 4.3 Neck Stretching Instructions to Relieve Nontraumatic, Primary Headache

1. Stretch your neck slowly through its range of motion
   - First bend your chin to your chest
   - Then turn your chin so it is touching your left shoulder
   - Then turn your chin to touch the right shoulder
   - Move your chin back to your chest and lift your chin up toward the ceiling
   - Repeat three to five times
2. Tip your left ear toward the left shoulder
   - Place your left hand on the right side of your head and press down gently to feel a stretch on the right side of your neck
   - Hold for 5 s. Then relax and repeat three times
   - Repeat for the other side by tipping your right ear toward your right shoulder and pressing your head gently to stretch the left side of your neck
3. Change your posture
   - Lie flat on a firm surface or ED stretcher and remove the pillows
   - Place a stack of books about 1–2 in. high behind your head. Position the books so that they are behind the top and middle of your head, leaving your neck free (see photo)
   - Relax in this position and feel your head move up slightly from your neck

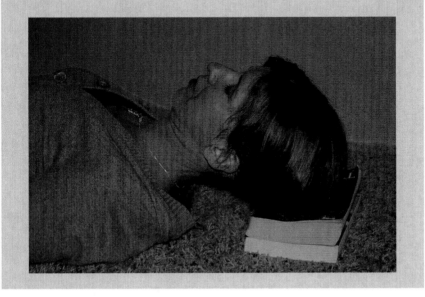

Selecting Medications for Headache in the ED

Despite the range of medications options for ED headache treatment, a prospective survey of adults seen in the ED for nontraumatic headache reported that 34% received neither any medication nor intravenous fluid [20]. Patients who were treated were most commonly prescribed anti-emetics or opioids. Two in every three patients had self-medicated prior to the ED visit, usually with nonopioid analgesics (77%). Only 6% had used a headache-specific treatment, such as dihydroergotamine (DHE) or a triptan. Therefore, pre-ED medications would not have precluded additional treatment in most cases.

Migraines in the ED are most effectively treated with anti-emetics and migraine-specific therapy, such as ergotamines and triptans. These effective migraine therapies are often dramatically underutilized in the ED. A review of 490 ED patients treated with parenteral medication for benign headache in three centers reported migraine as the most common diagnosis (58%), followed by nonspecific headache (41%), and tension-type headache (1%) [21]. The most frequently used medications were opioids, which were prescribed for almost half of all patients (Table 4.2). A subanalysis of only those patients diagnosed with migraine similarly showed

Table 4.2 Most commonly used parenteral medications for benign headache in the ED (based on [21])

Drug	Percentage patients for whom each drug was prescribed
Analgesic	
Any opioid	48
Hydromorphone	6
Meperidine	36
Morphine	3
Other opioids	4
Ketorolac	26
Anti-emetic	
Prochlorperazine	46
Diphenhydramine	37
Promethazine	23
Hydroxyzine	13
Droperidol	8
Metoclopramide	4
Migraine-specific drugs	
Dihydroergotamine	8
Sumatriptan	3
Glucocorticoids	
Dexamethasone	1
Methylprednisolone	0.5

Most patients received two medications (82%), with 24% receiving at least three parenteral medications, and 7% treated with at least four parenteral drugs

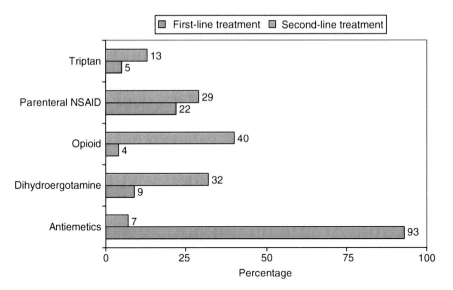

Fig. 4.4 Preferred treatment of migraine by ED practitioners (based on [5]). More than one drug could be identified as first- or second-line therapy. Second-line treatments were used when headache failed to improve with first-line treatment. *NSAID* non-steroidal anti-inflammatory drug

infrequent use of migraine-specific agents (DHE in 6% and sumatriptan in 3%), with anti-emetics used for 49%, opioids for 44%, and ketorolac for 16%. A subsequent survey asking 105 ED physicians and physician assistants to identify first- and second-line ED treatment for migraine reported anti-emetics and parenteral nonsteroidal anti-inflammatory drugs to be preferred first-line therapy, with opioids the preferred second-line treatment for patients failing first-line treatment (Fig. 4.4) [5]. Curiously, only a small minority of clinicians endorsed migraine-specific agents as first-line treatment (DHE 9%; triptans 5%). The primary reasons for selecting anti-emetics or nonopioid analgesics as first-line therapy were treatment efficacy, drug availability in the ED, clinicians having received training in using these medications, and conformity with ED practice patterns.

> **Pearl for the practitioner:**
> Migraine-specific medications underutilized in the ED.

Choosing Medications for Primary Headache

A prospective survey of 184 patients seen in an ED for primary headache (78% migraine, 22% tension-type) showed that both headache types were typically treated with the same medications [22]. This underscores the current thinking that migraine

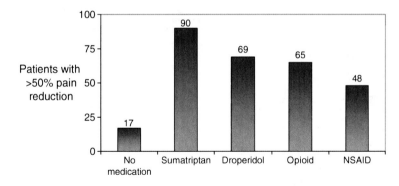

Fig. 4.5 Reduction in primary headache pain with ED treatment (based on [22])

and tension-type headaches may not be distinct headache types, but rather may represent two ends of a spectrum of headaches mediated by neurotransmitters like serotonin and dopamine. Among patients treated with medications, pain was reduced by more than half in 64% of patients. Patients treated with sumatriptan or droperidol experienced the greatest pain relief (Fig. 4.5), however, most patients given medications were initially treated with opioids (46%), with 26% receiving droperidol, 20% a nonsteroidal anti-inflammatory drug, and only 7% sumatriptan. Preferentially selecting dopamine-blocking anti-emetics or serotonergic headache-specific medications (e.g., triptans and dihydroergotamine) for primary headache rather than general analgesics may improve treatment outcome, especially for more severely impaired patients. Furthermore, selecting treatments with fewer sedating effects (e.g., sumatriptan and DHE) can help facilitate return to work or other daily activities.

Migraine

Migraine may be effectively treated in the ED with anti-emetics, migraine therapies (e.g., triptans, ergotamines, or valproate), or analgesics (e.g., nonsteroidal anti-inflammatory drugs) (see Table 4.3 and Fig. 4.6). Despite the availability of effective migraine treatment options, a retrospective survey of ED visits for migraine showed that most patients are treated with anti-emetics or analgesics [23]. Patients most commonly received intravenous treatment with prochlorperazine (61%), ketorolac (42%), or opioids (40%). Interestingly, half of the patients were not candidates for using a triptan due to using a triptan or ergotamine within the prevtious 24 h (28%), having a contraindicated medical condition (e.g., hypertension, cerebrovascular disease, cardiovascular disease, or pregnancy; 17%), or reporting an allergy to triptans or ergotamines (5%). Among the remaining half of patients who were eligible for migraine-specific therapy, only 12% received a migraine treatment. Benefits of using migraine-specific therapy rather than opioids include better efficacy, less sedation, and less potential for abuse/addiction.

Table 4.3 Typical non-anti-emetic medications for acute migraine

Drug	Dosing	Special instructions
Sumatriptan	4–6 mg SQ May also be given as two 3-mg doses separated by about 20 min	Avoid in patients with uncontrolled hypertension or cardiovascular disease. Transient chest and neck pressure and tightness are common and usually not associated with cardiac pathology. Avoid in patients using another triptan or DHE during the previous 24 h
Dihydroergotamine (DHE)	0.5 mg IV over 2–3 min; repeated in 1 h if needed	Avoid in patients with uncontrolled hypertension or cardiovascular disease. Premedicate with anti-emetic, e.g., ondansetron 8 mg IM or IV; metoclopramide 10 mg plus diphenhydramine 25 mg IV; or prochlorperazine 10 mg plus diphenhydramine 25 mg IV. Avoid in patients using triptan or ergotamine during the previous 24 h
Ketorolac	60 mg IM 30 mg IV	Avoid in patients with active peptic ulcer disease, coagulopathy, or patients with kidney disease (e.g., GFR <60 mL/min)
Valproate	300–500 mg IV drip administered slowly over 30 min	Avoid in patients who are pregnant or not using reliable contraception or patients with liver disease. Use cautiously if at all in patients using topiramate 50 mg daily or higher dosing
Magnesium	1 g IV over 20 min	Generally well tolerated

GFR glomerular filtration rate, *IM* intramuscular, *IV* intravenous, *SQ* subcutaneous

The European Federation of Neurological Societies task force recently published revised recommendations for emergency migraine treatment [24]. They recommend initial treatment with analgesic plus anti-emetic, with subcutaneous sumatriptan as an alternative therapy (Table 4.4). Studies detailing ED response for a variety of possible treatments are described below.

Triptans

Subcutaneous sumatriptan is an effective and well-tolerated treatment for primary headache. A prospective study evaluated outcome of 147 patients with primary headache (88% migraine and 12% tension-type headache) treated with 6 mg sumatriptan subcutaneously [25]. Half of all patients experienced a significant reduction in symptoms after 30 min, with a response in nearly 60% after 1 h (Fig. 4.7). One in three patients required additional therapy after 1 h, most commonly an anti-emetic or opioid. Response was similar for patients with either migraine or tension-type headache.

Side effects with subcutaneous sumatriptan often include pressure over the chest and neck [26]. While these side effects rarely signify cardiac pathology, triptan

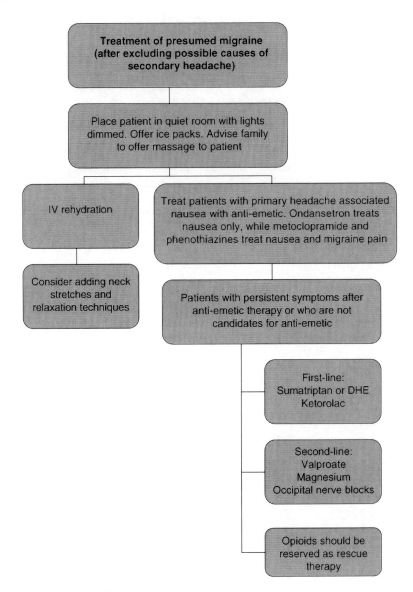

Fig. 4.6 Treatment algorithm

Table 4.4 European Federation of Neurological Societies recommendations for ED migraine treatment [24]

Treatment category	Treatment recommendation
First-line therapy	Intravenous administration of 1,000 mg aspirin with or without metoclopramide
	Subcutaneous sumatriptan 6 mg
Severe migraine treatment option	Dihydroergotamine 2 mg nasal spray or suppository
Prolonged migraine (>72 h)	50–100 mg prednisone
	10 mg dexamethasone

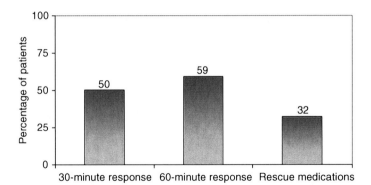

Fig. 4.7 ED response to primary headache treatment with sumatriptan [25]. Graph shows percentage of patients experiencing a reduction in headache severity of at least 50% and the percentage of patients using any rescue medication after 60 min

administration can result in mild and transient increases in blood pressure and effects on coronary artery tone [27]. Consequently, these drugs are contraindicated in patients with uncontrolled hypertension, cardiac ischemia, or other significant cardiovascular disease. Using a lower dose of sumatriptan (e.g., 4 mg subcutaneously) may also provide good migraine efficacy while minimizing unpleasant side effects [28]. Another option is to administer 3 mg subcutaneously, wait for 20 min, and then administer a second 3 mg dose.

> **Pearl for the practitioner:**
> Although sumatriptan has been administered intravenously in research studies, it is not used intravenously in clinical treatment.

Ergotamine

DHE is well established as a successful acute therapy for severe migraine episodes, with a prolonged duration of action that helps limit recurrence among patients with typically long-lasting attacks. Intramuscular DHE 1 mg was tested against 1.5 mg/kg meperidine in a randomized, double-blind study of adults with acute migraine in the ED (Fig. 4.8) [29]. Both groups received concomitant therapy with the antihistamine hydroxyzine (Vistaril). Patients receiving either treatment experienced similar improvement in migraine symptoms, although recurrence was more common in patients receiving meperidine.

MAP0004 [Levadex] is a novel, orally inhaled formulation of DHE shown to be effective in the treatment of acute migraine [15] with fewer adverse events compared with intravenous DHE dosing [16]. MAP0004, currently under review by the FDA, may be a useful option to reduce side effects from DHE and for patients without venous access.

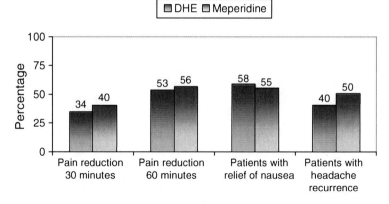

Fig. 4.8 Intramuscular DHE vs. meperidine for ED migraine in adults (based on [29])

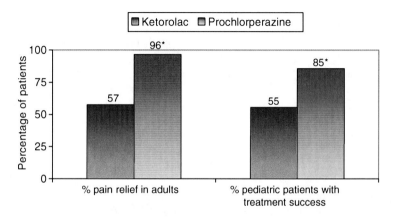

Fig. 4.9 ED treatment with ketorolac vs. prochlorperazine (based on [30] and [31]). All patients were randomly assigned to double-blind intravenous treatment with ketorolac (30 mg in adults and 0.5 mg/kg to a maximum dose of 30 mg in children) or prochlorperazine (10 mg in adults or 0.15 mg/kg to a maximum dose of 10 mg). Successful treatment in children was defined as headache reduction of at least 50%. Numerical differences were significant (*$P < 0.05$)

Nonopioid Analgesics

Intravenous ketorolac is an effective nonopioid ED option for severe headache; however, controlled studies consistently show inferior efficacy compared with anti-emetics when treating migraine in either adults or children (Fig. 4.9) [30, 31]. Intravenous ketorolac did result in superior reduction in migraine pain in adults randomized to 30 mg ketorolac vs. 20 mg intranasal sumatriptan (77% vs. 27%, $P < 0.05$) [32].

Pearl for the practitioner:
Intramuscular or intravenous ketorolac is a safe, well-tolerated option for treating acute headache.

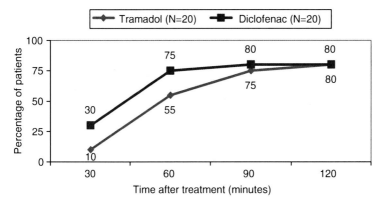

Fig. 4.10 Percentage of patients experiencing pain relief after ED migraine treatment with intramuscular tramadol or nonsteroidal anti-inflammatory drug diclofenac (based on [34]). None of the numerical differences was statistically significant

Some patients may also benefit from tramadol. A slow infusion of 100 mg tramadol in 100 mL saline vs. placebo in a single-blind, randomized study resulted in significantly better pain relief after 1 h than placebo (71% vs. 35%, $P<0.05$) [33]. Headache recurrence was similar for both groups. Fig. 4.10 shows pain reduction in adults seeking ED treatment for migraine after being randomized to double-blind, intramuscular treatment with 100 mg tramadol or 75 mg diclofenac [34]. Response occurred earlier with diclofenac. Two-hour reductions in headache, photophobia, phonophobia, and nausea were similar with either treatment. Rescue treatment at 2 h was used by 20% of patients receiving either treatment.

Valproate

Intravenous valproate offers an effective alternative acute migraine treatment in patients who are not pregnant and are using adequate contraception. Patients must be explicitly asked about the chance of pregnancy and whether they are using a reliable form of contraception, with this information documented in the chart prior to using valproate. A small study treated 40 migraine patients intravenously with 500 mg valproate vs. 10 mg prochlorperazine, each diluted in 10 mL saline and administered over 2 min [35]. Efficacy was better with prochlorperazine, with additional rescue therapy required in 79% treated with valproate vs. 25% with prochlorperazine.

In an open-label study, acute migraine patients were randomized to receive intravenous valproate or intramuscular DHE with metoclopramide [36]. One hour after treatment, pain and nausea decreased with both treatments although photophobia and phonophobia persisted (Fig. 4.11). While early treatment response was similar, sustained relief was better with DHE with metoclopramide. Twenty-four hours after treatment, a moderate to severe headache was reported by 40% with valproate

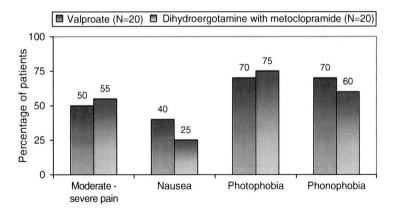

Fig. 4.11 Migraine symptoms reported 1 h post-treatment with valproate or dihydroergotamine plus metoclopramide (based on [58]).These numerical differences were not tested for statistical significance. Outcome was compared 4-h after treatment, with no significant between-treatment differences

and 10% with dihydroergotamine with metoclopramide. None of the valproate-treated patients reported medication side effects, while 15% of the dihydroergotamine with metoclopramide group reported nausea and diarrhea during the first 4 h after treatment.

Valproate can interact with topiramate to produce delirium/encephalopathy thought to be related to a hyperammonemic state [37, 38]. It is the opinion of the authors that valproate should not be given if the patient is taking more than 50 mg daily of topiramate, though some clinicians use this combination with cautious monitoring.

> ***Pearl for the practitioner:***
> Intravenous valproate 500 mg administered over 2 min is an option for acute migraine, but generally should not be given to patients treated with daily doses of topiramate ≥50 mg.

Magnesium

Intravenous magnesium sulfate may also be used in the ED treatment of migraine, with efficacy shown with 1 g intravenously [39]. In a randomized, prospective study, 2 g intravenous magnesium sulfate was as effective as 10 mg intravenous metoclopramide and more effective than placebo [40].

> ***Pearl for the practitioner:***
> Intravenous magnesium 1–2 g is an effective option for acute migraine.

Steroids

Corticosteroids offer limited benefit for acute migraine treatment. Dexamethasone has minimal efficacy in most patients receiving ED treatment of migraine, although benefit has been shown in patients with migraine lasting >72 h [41]. Double-blind, placebo-controlled studies have evaluated the benefit of adjunctive steroid treatment to reduce headache recurrence after treatment in the ED. Treatment with either oral or intravenous dexamethasone failed to reduce migraine recurrence [42–45].

> ***Pearl for the practitioner:***
> Corticosteroids have shown inconsistent benefit for treating ED headache. 10 mg IV dexamethasone may be helpful in the ED for patients reporting migraine lasting >72 h.

Octreotide

Somatostatin mimic octreotide (Sandostatin) inhibits neuroactive substances important in migraine pathogenesis (e.g., serotonin, bradykinin, substance P, and prostaglandins) and has been shown to reduce the severity of acute migraine [46]. Octreotide has recently been tested for migraine treatment in the ED [47]. In a small, double-blind, placebo-controlled study, 44 patients were randomized to receive 100 µg octreotide or 10 mg prochlorperazine administered intravenously over 2 min. Pain relief was superior with prochlorperazine (71% reduction in pain with prochlorperazine vs. 44% reduction with octreotide, $P=0.03$), with rescue therapy needed after 1 h in 48% of octreotide patients and 10% treated with prochlorperazine ($P<0.01$). Headache recurred in 48–72 h for 25% with octreotide and 10% with prochlorperazine. Akathisia occurred more commonly among patients treated with prochlorperazine (35% vs. 9%, $P<0.01$).

Opioid Analgesics

While opioid analgesics are widely used for headache treatment in the ED, their efficacy as headache-relieving treatment is inferior to most previously discussed medications. Despite the fact that opioids offer only modest benefit for migraine relief, a survey of 500 randomly selected ED charts from patients with a primary diagnosis of migraine showed opioids to be the most commonly prescribed first-line ED treatment (60% of patients) [48]. The reasons for the widespread use of opioids in the

ED is unclear, but may be related to the unfamiliarity of patients and providers with headache-specific medications relative to their comfort with opioids. Furthermore, many of the opioid medications produce euphoric, anxiolytic, and sedating properties, which may make them more desirable for patients seeking nonanalgesic drug properties. Caution should be exercised when administering potential medications of abuse like opioids. Self-report of ongoing problems with substances of abuse are often unreliable. In one survey, 17% of patients seeking opioid treatment in the ED for headache tested positive on urine screens for drugs of abuse that they failed to report they had taken [49]. Identified substances were benzodiazepines, marijuana, and cocaine. Routinely treating headaches with opioids can encourage drug-seeking behavior [50]. Furthermore, a recent study showed that migraine patients treated with opioids in the ED had longer duration visits compared with patients treated with nonopioids, further supporting cautious use in patients with benign headache [51].

Opioids are most appropriately used as rescue rather than first-line headache treatment. When parenteral opioids are used, avoid meperidine because of potential risks with accumulation of metabolites, such as normeperidine. Some ED physicians prefer to avoid short-acting opioids, such as meperidine and hydromorphone, in favor of the longer acting opioids, such as nalbuphine (Nubain), if they are used at all (personal communication with Merle Diamond, MD).

Cluster Headache

Cluster headache is quite short-lived and will typically not present to the ED. Cluster headache episodes, though intensely severe, will generally resolve spontaneously within 60–90 min, often before many potential treatments would be expected to start taking effect. The primary focus for cluster headache in the ED is establishing the diagnosis, beginning transitional preventive therapy to minimize repeated episodes, and connecting the patients with close follow-up with headache-interested providers. Acute therapies may be offered to patients experiencing a cluster attack during the ED visit.

100% Oxygen

Patients with cluster headache who report to the ED with an acute attack may be treated with 100% oxygen at 8–12 L/min by face mask. A recent double-blind, placebo-controlled study provided data for 76 cluster headache patients randomly treating four attacks with 100% oxygen 12 L/min by face mask or air for 15 min at the onset of each attack (Fig. 4.12) [52]. Complete relief of cluster headache pain after 15 min was achieved by 78% with oxygen vs. 20% with air placebo ($P < 0.001$). While 100% oxygen may lessen the severity of an acute attack, it will not prevent subsequent episodes from occurring.

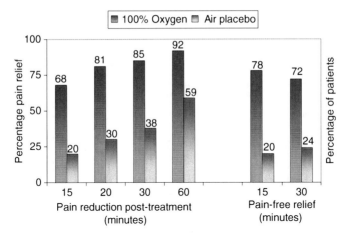

Fig. 4.12 Cluster headache relief with oxygen (based on [52])

Table 4.5 Cluster headache relief with triptans (based on [53])

Acute treatment	Headache relief in 30 min		
	Triptan (%)	Placebo (%)	NNT 30-min
Zolmitriptan 5 mg nasal spray	45	26	5.2
Zolmitriptan 10 mg nasal spray	62	26	2.8
Sumatriptan 20 mg nasal spray	57	26	NR
	Headache relief in 15 min		
	Triptan (%)	Placebo (%)	NNT 15-min
Zolmitriptan 5 mg nasal spray	15	7	12
Zolmitriptan 10 mg nasal spray	28	7	4.9
Sumatriptan 6 mg SQ	75	32	2.4

NNT number of patients needing treatment for one patient to achieve headache relief,
NR not reported

Triptans

Intranasal and injectable triptans may also be used for acute treatment of cluster headache, although efficacy is generally less than that seen with migraine (Table 4.5) [53]. Because of the short duration of cluster headaches, fast-acting parenteral triptans are the most effective, with intranasal preparations having intermediate efficacy and oral preparations being the least effective.

Other Acute Therapies

Performing on occipital nerve block with 2.5 mL 0.5% bupivacaine and 20 mg methylprednisolone on the side of the cluster pain has also been shown to effectively relieve cluster headache pain [54] (see instructions below).

Intranasal lidocaine may be a useful rescue therapy in patients failing to achieve relief of their cluster attack with other therapies [55]. The patient should be instructed to put 0.5–1 mL (10–20 drops) of 4% viscous lidocaine in the ipsilateral nostril while lying flat on the back with the head hanging over the side of the bed. Treatment can be repeated once, if needed, after 2 min.

> ***Pearl for the practitioner:***
> Effective treatments for acute cluster headache include
>
> - 100% O_2 7–12 L/min by face mask
> - Sumatriptan 6 mg subcutaneous injection
> - Zolmitriptan 5 or 10 mg nasal spray
> - Sumatriptan 20 mg nasal spray
> - Occipital nerve block

Transitional Prevention Therapies

If patients are well into their current cluster period and experiencing several headaches each day, they may be candidates for short-term transitional corticosteroid therapy to help break the cluster cycle, e.g., prednisone 10–60 mg/day for 1 week or an occipital nerve block (see below) [55]. Furthermore, follow-up with a primary care or other headache-interested provider should be arranged ideally within 24 h of the ED visit for cluster headache to consider additional maintenance preventive therapy, e.g., verapamil, topiramate, or lithium.

Anesthetic Therapy

Trigger point injections are most often used to treat recalcitrant tension-type headache, while occipital nerve blocks are most commonly performed to treat occipital neuralgia and chronic migraine [56]. Both types of injections can provide temporary pain relief that can augment other headache treatments.

Trigger Point Injections

Myofascial trigger points are more than simply tender areas. A trigger point is a tender area within contracted muscle bands that produces an involuntary contraction

Fig. 4.13 Referral pattern
for upper trapezius trigger
points [reprinted with
permission. Marcus DA.
Chronic pain. A primary care
guide to practical
management. 2nd ed. New
York: Humana Press; 2009.]

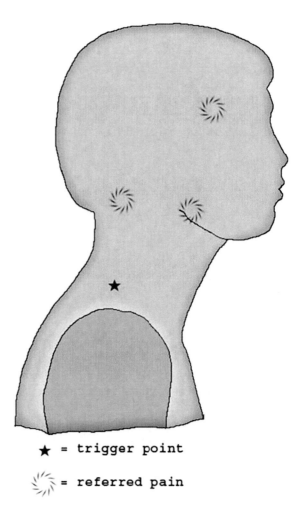

★ = trigger point

= referred pain

with stimulation, such as physically plucking or inserting a needle into the muscle
[57]. Trigger points may be locally tender (called *latent trigger points*) or they
may refer pain to predictable areas (called *active trigger points*). For example,
active trigger points in the upper trapezius characteristically refer pain to the head
(Fig. 4.13).

Trigger point injections require infiltration with a local anesthetic into myofascial
trigger points. A procedure summary is provided in Box 4.4. In most cases, steroids
do not need to be included in trigger point injections as it is not clear that the addition
of steroids lengthens the duration of pain relief. Trigger point injections are
contraindicated in patients with a risk for coagulopathy or bleeding.

Box 4.4 Trigger Point Injection Procedure

- Insert a 22- to 25-gauge needle into the skin, approximately 1 cm away from the trigger point
- Advance the needle to the trigger point
- Verify the needle has been placed outside of blood vessels by gently drawing back on the syringe and noting the absence of blood
- Inject 0.1–0.2 mL of local anesthetic
- Partially withdraw the needle, redirect, and advance toward another area within the trigger point
- Repeat this process until one of the following three conditions has been met:
  - A local twitch response is no longer elicited
  - Muscle tautness is reduced
  - 0.5–1.0 mL of anesthetic has been injected around the trigger point
- Withdraw the needle and maintain pressure over the injected area to minimize hematoma development

Trigger points may also be effectively treated using superficial dry needling, which involves inserting a solid thin needle (resembling an acupuncture needle) into the trigger point. This method can also help deactivate myofascial trigger points when used in conjunction with stretching exercises [58]. In patients with trigger points, dry needling results in significantly reduced pain and improved range of motion [59]. The benefits of dry needling are further supported by studies showing similar benefits after trigger point injections, regardless of the injected substance (including saline) [60].

Occipital Nerve Blocks

Occipital nerve blocks effectively treat migraine in about half of consecutively treated patients [61, 62]. In one series, unilateral greater occipital nerve blocks resulted in prolonged pain relief benefits [62]. In this series, each block used a 3-mL mixture of 2% lidocaine and 80 mg of methylprednisolone. Complete or partial pain relief was achieved by 46% of migraine patients. Most patients experienced complete relief for 7 days, with a mean duration of relief of 20 days. Partial response lasted for 20 days in most patients, with a mean duration of partial response of 45 days. Pretreatment tenderness over the greater occipital nerve predicted success. Furthermore, as noted above, greater occipital nerve blocks can occasionally be an effective transitional option for patients in active cluster.

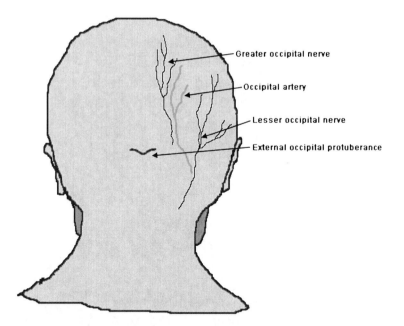

Greater occipital nerve

Occipital artery

Lesser occipital nerve

External occipital protuberance

Fig. 4.14 Occipital nerve anatomy [reprinted with permission. Marcus, Bain. Effective migraine treatment in pregnant and lactating women. A practical guide. New York: Humana Press; 2009]

Anatomic studies show the greater occipital nerve is generally located, on average, 22% of the distance between the external occipital protuberance and the mastoid process (Fig. 4.14) [63]. The nerve is, therefore, typically located about 2 cm (about 2 finger breadths) lateral to the external occipital protuberance [63]. Figure 4.15 shows the preparation tray and the procedure, which are described in Boxes 4.5 and 4.6.

Other Injections

Intramuscular injections of 1.5 mL of 0.5% bupivacaine bilateral to the sixth or seventh cervical vertebra were found to benefit patients seeking ED treatment for headache in a retrospective review of 417 patients [64]. Bupivacaine was slowly injected using a 1.5-in. 25-gauge needle inserted 1–1.5 in. into the paraspinous musculature 2–3 cm bilateral to the spinous process of the sixth or seventh cervical vertebrae (Fig. 4.16). Most patients responded to treatment (Fig. 4.17), with alternative headache therapies generally initiated within 20–30 min for patients experiencing inadequate or incomplete pain relief.

Fig. 4.15 Occipital nerve
block procedure. (**a**) The
preparation tray. (**b**) The head
has been marked to show
probable location of the
occipital nerves

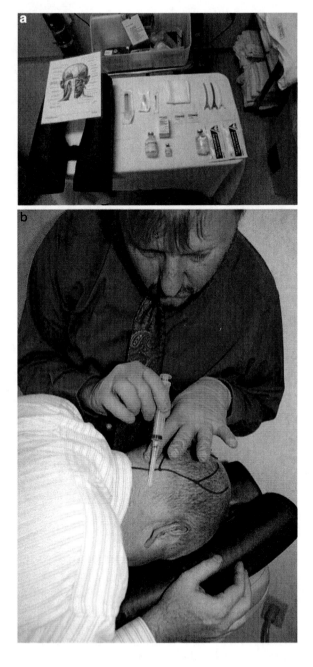

Box 4.5 Occipital Nerve Block Prep Tray

- 10 mL syringe
- 18-Ga 1½ in. needle
- 25-Ga 1½ in. needle
- 1% xylocaine without epinephrine
- 8.4% $NaHCO_3$ buffering solution
- Triamcinalone acetonide 10 mg/1 mL corticosteroid solution
- Alcohol wipes
- Povidone-iodine topical antiseptic swabs (e.g., Betadine)
- 4×4 gauze pads
- Sterile gloves
- Clips to hold back long hair
- Anatomical drawing
- Massage pillow

Box 4.6 Performing an Occipital Nerve Block

- Indication
  - Greater and/or lesser occipital nerve region pain
- Preprocedure explanation: Describe the procedure to the patient and obtain informed consent
  - Use anatomical drawing to illustrate the procedure
  - Review patient medical problems, medications, and allergies
  - Review common risks of infection, numbness, and bleeding
- Performing the block
  - Ask the patient to lie prone, using the massage pillow if available
  - Clean an area 2 finger breadths lateral to the midline occipital protuberance. Wash both sides if the procedure is intended to be done bilaterally
  - Draw up 3 mL of 1% lidocaine plus 0.5 mL of 8.4% $NaHCO_3$ buffering solution plus 1 mL of the kenalog 10 mg/mL solution using the 18-Ga 1½ in. needle. If the procedure will be done bilaterally, double the amount of each of the above solutions
  - Ask the patient to begin to focus on her breathing, taking deep breaths in through the nose and exhaling out through the mouth
  - Stand on the opposite side from where the injection will be given
  - With a sterile, gloved hand, palpate the proposed entry sight 2 finger breadths lateral to the midline occipital protuberance. If the area is tender, this predicts a more favorable response

(continued)

Box 4.6 (continued)

- Using the 25-Ga 1½ in. needle, aim for the mid-helix injecting away from the midline
- After ensuring the needle is outside of any blood vessels, inject approximately ⅓ of the 5 mL solution
- Withdraw the needle and redirect it toward the top of the helix, ensure placement, and inject approximately ⅓ of the 5 mL solution
- Finally, withdraw the needle and redirect it toward the ear lobe, ensure placement, and inject the remaining ⅓ of the 5 mL solution
- After the needle is withdrawn, repeat the procedure on the contralateral side, if the area is tender, using the same procedure after moving to the opposite side of the patient and injecting away from the midline again
- When the procedure is finished, massage the medication into the scalp for 3–5 min

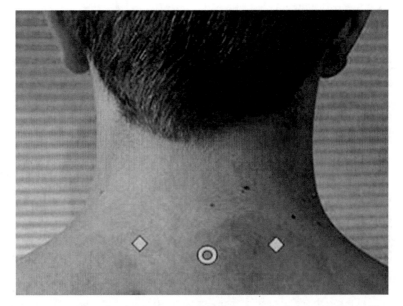

Fig. 4.16 Location for performing lower cervical bupivacaine injections (reproduced with permission from [64]). The lower cervical injections are performed in the paraspinous muscles bilateral to the C6 or C7 spinous process. The injections are performed at a distance of approximately 2–3 cm from the spinous process. The spinous process is marked here with a circle and the injection sites with diamonds

Fig. 4.17 Relief after lower
cervical vertebrae
bupivacaine injections
(based on [64])

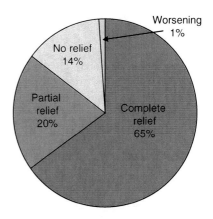

Deciding If Treatment Is Helpful

Prior to initiating treatment, patients are generally asked to gauge the severity of symptoms, such as pain, photophobia, and nausea, using a zero to ten-point scale, with zero representing no symptoms and ten excruciating/disabling symptoms. Symptomatic reduction of several points to more moderate severity symptoms is generally considered to represent effective treatment in clinical practice as these numeric rating scales are easy for patients to understand and the staff to interpret.

A variety of endpoints have been used in research to help define benefits from ED treatment of migraine. Commonly used endpoints include reductions in pain and disability (Table 4.6) [65]. A newly proposed, clinically practical, and patient-driven endpoint is to ask patients *would you take this treatment again?* This variable correlated with the other individual outcome measures and researchers speculated that this simple question might provide a more complete picture of the patient's migraine relief experience than focusing exclusively on pain, disability, or treatment side effects alone. Consequently, this might be an important question to ask and document in the chart, so that these data are available if the patient later returns for the treatment of a similar headache episode.

> ***Pearl for the practitioner:***
> An effective measure of migraine relief is to ask patients, "*Would you take this treatment again?*"

Table 4.6 Common endpoints for migraine relief in the ED (based on [65])

Endpoint	Time after treatment when typically assessed (h)
Reduction of migraine pain to mild severity	1 or 2
Reduction in pain by 33–90%	2
Complete relief of migraine pain	1 or 2
Relief of functional disability	2
Sustained relief of migraine	24

Reducing Headache Recurrence

Up to three in four patients treated in the ED for headache report recurrence of headache within 48 h of ED discharge [66]. The benefits of adding steroids to ED migraine treatment to reduce recurrence remain controversial, with studies providing conflicting results. While several individual, randomized, controlled studies failed to identify benefit when adding intravenous or oral dexamethasone or oral prednisone to ED treatment for reducing recurrence [42, 67, 68], data pooled from seven clinical trials did show a moderate and statistically significant risk reduction of 9.7% when dexamethasone was added to usual ED migraine care [69]. In other words, for every 1,000 migraine patients treated in the ED with usual migraine treatments, adding dexamethasone would be expected to prevent recurrence of moderate to severe headache within 24–72 h after discharge from the ED in 97 patients. Interestingly, six of the seven included trials had failed to show efficacy benefits, suggesting low sample sizes may have contributed to the lack of observed significant response in individual trials. Using the pooled data for those trials reporting side effects, adverse events occurred for 26% treated with dexamethasone vs. 23% with placebo. Anecdotally, a short course of prednisone (20 mg twice daily for 5 days) has been found to be helpful.

> **Pearl for the practitioner:**
> A short course of steroids (e.g., prednisone 20 mg twice daily for 5 days) at discharge is sometime helpful for reducing migraine recurrence.

Because recurrence is relatively common, it is crucial for the ED provider to make sure that the patient has close follow-up with a headache-interested provider as well as a clear written protocol for interim treatment to prevent unnecessary repeat ED visits. More specific information about arranging follow-up care and providing an effective interim treatment strategy is provided in Chap. 9.

Summary

- Treat dehydration aggressively; most patients with severe headache will need intravenous rehydration.
- Anti-emetics (e.g., prochlorperazine and metoclopramide) are preferred first-line ED migraine treatment, effectively relieving both headache-related pain and nausea in ED migraine. Ondansetron may be used for nausea relief, although additional therapy will be needed to reduce other headache symptoms, such as pain.

- Patients treated with metoclopramide or phenothiazines should be monitored for akathisia and other extrapyramidal effects. Pretreatment with diphenhydramine may minimize the development of these side effects.
- Studies show that anti-emetics like metoclopramide or phenothiazines generally work as well as subcutaneous sumatriptan and better than opioids for ED migraine.
- Including nondrug pain-relieving therapies, trigger point injections, and occipital nerve blocks for appropriate patients can augment the ED treatment armamentarium.
- Subcutaneous sumatriptan, DHE, and nonopioid analgesics may also be used for nontraumatic, primary headache in the ED.
- ED providers should be able to diagnose patients with cluster headache accurately, treat the acute pain if it is still present in the ED, provide a transitional strategy, and arrange close follow-up with a headache-interested provider.

References

1. Wöber C, Wöber-Bingöl C. Triggers of migraine and tension-type headache. Handb Clin Neurol. 2010;97:161–72.
2. Blau JN. Water deprivation: a new migraine precipitant. Headache. 2005;45:757–9.
3. Martins IP, Gouveia RG. More on water and migraine. Cephalalgia. 2007;27:372–4.
4. Spigt MG, Kuijper EC, Schayck CP, et al. Increasing daily water intake for prophylactic treatment of headache: a pilot trial. Eur J Neurol. 2005;12:715–8.
5. Hurtado TR, Vinson DR, Vandenberg JT. ED treatment of migraine headache: factors influencing pharmacotherapeutic choices. Headache. 2007;47:1134–43.
6. Kelly AM, Walcynski T, Gunn B. The relative efficacy of phenothiazines for the treatment of acute migraine: a meta-analysis. Headache. 2009;49:1324–32.
7. Friedman BW, Esses D, Solorzano C, et al. A randomized controlled trial of prochlorperazine versus metoclopramide for treatment of acute migraine. Ann Emerg Med. 2008;52:399–406.
8. Miner JR, Fish SJ, Smith SW, Biros MH. Droperidol vs. prochlorperazine for benign headaches in the emergency department. Acad Emerg Med. 2001;8:873–9.
9. Richman PB, Allegra J, Eskin B, et al. A randomized clinical trial to assess the efficacy of intramuscular droperidol for the treatment of acute migraine. Am J Emerg Med. 2002;20:39–42.
10. Dusitanond P, Young WB. Neuroleptics and migraine. Cent Nerv Syst Agents Med Chem. 2009;9:63–70.
11. Ayad RF, Assar MD, Simpson L, Garner JB, Schussler JM. Causes and management of drug-induced QT syndrome. Proc (Baylor Univ Med Cent). 2010;23:250–5.
12. Keller GA, Ponte ML, Di Girolamo G. Other drugs acting on nervous system associated with QT-interval prolongation. Curr Drug Saf. 2010;5:105–11.
13. Dusitanond P, Young WB. Neuroleptics and migraine. Cent Nerv Syst Agents Med Chem. 2009;9:63–70.
14. Griffith JD, Mycyck MB, Kyriacou DN. Metoclopramide versus hydrocodone for the emergency department treatment of migraine headache. J Pain. 2008;9:88–94.
15. Cicek M, Karcioglu O, Pariak I, et al. Prospective, randomized, double-blind, controlled comparison of metoclopramide and pethidine in the emergency treatment of acute primary vascular and tension-type headache episodes. Emerg Med J. 2004;21:323–6.
16. Friedman BW, Corbo J, Lipton RB. A trial of metoclopramide vs sumatriptan for the emergency department treatment of migraines. Neurology. 2005;64:463–8.

17. Friedman BW, Hockberg M, Esses D, et al. A clinical trial of trimethobenzamide/diphenhydramine versus sumatriptan for acute migraine. Headache. 2006;46:934–41.
18. Kostic MA, Gutierrez FJ, Rieg TS, Moore TS, Gendrom RT. A prospective, randomized trial of intravenous prochlorperazine versus subcutaneous sumatriptan in acute migraine therapy in the emergency department. Ann Emerg Med. 2010;56:1–6.
19. Dillard JN, Knapp S. Complementary and alternative pain therapy in the emergency department. Emerg Med Clin N Am. 2005;23:529–49.
20. Gupta MX, Silberstein SD, Young WB, et al. Less is not more: underutilization of headache medications in a university hospital emergency department. Headache. 2007;47:1125–33.
21. Vinson DR, Hurtado TR, Vandenberg JT, Banwart L. Variations among emergency departments in the treatment of benign headache. Ann Emerg Med. 2003;41:90–7.
22. Trainor A, Miner J. Pain treatment and relief among patients with primary headache subtypes in the ED. Am J Emerg. 2008;26:1029–34.
23. Friedman D, Feldon S, Holloway R, Fisher S. Utilization, diagnosis, treatment and cost of migraine treatment in the emergency department. Headache. 2009;49:1163–73.
24. Evers A, Áfra J, Frese A, et al. EFNS guideline on the drug treatment of migraine – revised report of an EFNS task force. Eur J Neurol. 2009;16:968–81.
25. Miner JR, Smith SW, Moore J, Biros M. Sumatriptan for the treatment of undifferentiated primary headaches in the ED. Am J Emerg Med. 2007;25:60–4.
26. Visser WH, Jaspers NM, de Vriend RH, Ferrari MD. Chest symptoms after sumatriptan: a two-year clinical practice review in 735 consecutive migraine patients. Cephalalgia. 1996;16:554–9.
27. Martin VT, Goldstein JA. Evaluating the safety and tolerability profile of acute treatments for migraine. Am J Med. 2005;118(Suppl):36S–44S.
28. Wendt J, Cady R, Singer R, et al. A randomized, double-blind, placebo-controlled trial of the efficacy and tolerability of a 4-mg dose of subcutaneous sumatriptan for the treatment of acute migraine attacks in adults. Clin Ther. 2006;28:517–26.
29. Carleston SG, Shesser RF, Pietrzak MP, et al. Double-blind, multicenter trial to compare the efficacy of intramuscular dihydroergotamine plus hydroxyzine versus intramuscular meperidine plus hydroxyzine for the emergency department treatment of acute migraine headache. Ann Emerg Med. 1998;32:129–38.
30. Seim MB, March JA, Dunn KA. Intravenous ketorolac vs intravenous prochlorperazine for the treatment of migraine headaches. Acad Emerg Med. 1998;5:573–6.
31. Brousseau DC, Duffy SJ, Anderson AC, Linakis JG. Treatment of pediatric migraine headaches: a randomized, double-blind trial of prochlorperazine versus ketorolac. Ann Emerg Med. 2004;43:256–62.
32. Meredith JT, Wait S, Brewer KL. A prospective double-blind study of nasal sumatriptan versus IV ketorolac in migraine. Am J Emerg Med. 2003;21:173–5.
33. Alemdar M, Pekdemir M, Selekler HM. Single-dose intravenous tramadol for acute migraine pain in adults: a single-blind, prospective, randomized, placebo-controlled clinical trail. Clin Ther. 2007;29:1441–7.
34. Engindeniz Z, Demircan C, Karli N, et al. Intramuscular tramadol vs. diclofenac sodium for the treatment of acute migraine attacks in emergency department: a prospective, randomized, double-blind study. J Headache Pain. 2005;6:143–8.
35. Tanen DA, Miller S, French T, Riffenburgh RH. Intravenous sodium valproate versus prochlorperazine for the emergency department treatment of acute migraine headaches: a prospective, randomized, double-blind trial. Ann Emerg Med. 2003;41:847–53.
36. Edwards KR, Norton J, Behnke M. Comparison of intravenous valproate versus intramuscular dihydroergotamine and metoclopramide for acute treatment of migraine headaches. Headache. 2001;41:976–80.
37. Deutsch SI, Burket JA, Rosse RB. Valproate-induced hyperammonemic encephalopathy and normal liver functions: possible synergism with topiramate. Clin Neuropharmacol. 2009;32:350–2.

38. Vivekanandan S, Nayak SD. Valproate-induced hyperammonemic encephalopathy enhanced by topiramate and phenobarbitone: a case report and an update. Ann Indian Acad Neurol. 2010;13:145–7.
39. Bigal ME, Bordini CA, Tepper SJ, Speciali JG. Intravenous magnesium sulphate in the acute treatment of migraine without aura and migraine with aura. A randomized, double-blind, placebo-controlled study. Cephalalgia. 2002;22:345–53.
40. Cete Y, Dora B, Ertan C, Ozdemir C, Oktay C. A randomized prospective placebo-controlled study of intravenous magnesium sulphate vs. metoclopramide in the management of acute migraine attacks in the Emergency Department. Cephalalgia. 2005;25:199–204.
41. Friedman BW, Greenwald P, Bania TC, et al. Randomized trial of IV dexamethasone for acute migraine in the emergency department. Neurology. 2007;69:2038–44.
42. Kelly AM, Kerr D, Clooney M. Impact of oral dexamethasone versus placebo after ED treatment of migraine with phenothiazines on the rate of recurrent headache: a randomized controlled trial. Emerg Med J. 2008;25:26–9.
43. Friedman BW, Greenwald P. Bania, et al. Randomized trial of IV dexamethasone for acute migraine in the emergency department. Neurology. 2007;69:2038–44.
44. Rowe BH, Colman I, Edmonds ML, et al. Randomized controlled trial of intravenous dexamethasone to prevent relapse in acute migraine headache. Headache. 2008;28:333–40.
45. Donaldson D, Sundermann R, Jackson R, Bastani A. Intravenous dexamethasone vs placebo as adjunctive therapy to reduce the recurrence rate of acute migraine headaches: a multicenter, double-blind, placebo-controlled randomized clinical trial. Am J Emerg Med. 2008;26:124–30.
46. Kapicioğlu S, Gökce E, Kapicioğlu Z, Ovali E. Treatment of migraine attacks with a long-acting somatostatin analogue (octreotide, SMS 2010–995). Cephalalgia. 1997;17:27–30.
47. Miller MA, Levsky ME, Enslow W, Rosin A. Randomized evaluation of octreotide vs prochlorperazine for ED treatment of migraine headache. Am J Emerg Med. 2009;27:160–4.
48. Colman I, Rothney A, Wright SC, Zilkalns B, Rowe BH. Use of narcotic analgesics in the emergency department treatment of migraine headache. Neurology. 2004;62:1695–700.
49. Schuckman H, Hazelett S, Powell C, Steer S. A validation of self-reported substance use with biochemical testing among patients presenting to the emergency department seeking treatment for backache, headache, and toothache. Subst Use Misuse. 2008;43:589–95.
50. Braden JB, Russo J, Fan MY, et al. Emergency department visits among recipients of chronic opioid therapy. Arch Intern Med. 2010;170:1425–32.
51. Tornabene SV, Deutsch R, Davis DP, Chan TC, Vilke GM. Evaluating the use and timing of opioids for the treatment of migraine headaches in the emergency department. J Emerg Med. 2009;36:333–7.
52. Cohen AS, Burns B, Goadsby PJ. High-flow oxygen for treatment of cluster headache: a randomized trial. JAMA. 2009;302:2451–7.
53. Law S, Derry S, Moore RA. Triptans for acute cluster headache. Cochrane Database Syst Rev. 2010;4:CD008042.
54. May A, Leone M, Afra J, et al. EFNS Task Force. EFNS guidelines on the treatment of cluster headache and other trigeminal-autonomic cephalalgias. Eur J Neurol. 2006;13:1066–77.
55. Halker R, Vargas B, Dodick DW. Cluster headache: diagnosis and treatment. Semin Neurol. 2010;30:175–85.
56. Blumfeld A, Ashkenazi A, Grosberg B, et al. Patterns of use of peripheral nerve blocks and trigger point injections among headache practitioners in the USA: results of the American Headache Society Interventional Procedure Survey (AHS-IPS). Headache. 2010;50:937–42.
57. Simons DG, Travell JG, Simons LS. Myofascial pain and dysfunction: the trigger point manual, vol 1. 2nd ed. Baltimore: Lippincott Williams & Wilkins; 1999.
58. Edwards J, Knowles N. Superficial dry needling and active stretching in the treatment of myofascial pain – a randomized controlled trial. Acupunct Med. 2003;21:80–6.
59. Hsieh YL, Kao MJ, Kuan TS, et al. Dry needling to a key myofascial trigger point may reduce the irritability of satellite MTrPs. Am J Phys Med Rehabil. 2007;86(5):397–403.

60. Cummings TM, White AR. Needling therapies in the management of myofascial trigger point pain: a systematic review. Arch Phys Med Rehabil. 2001;82:986–92.
61. Weibelt S, Andress-Rothrock D, King W, Rothrock J. Suboccipital nerve blocks for suppression of chronic migraine: safety, efficacy, and predictors of outcome. Headache. 2010;50: 1041–4.
62. Afridi SK, Shields KG, Bhola R, Goadsby PJ. Greater occipital nerve injection in primary headache symptoms – prolonged effects from a single injection. Pain. 2006;122:126–9.
63. Loukas M, El-Sedfy A, Tubbs RS, et al. Identification of greater occipital nerve landmarks for the treatment of occipital neuralgia. Folia Morphol. 2006;65:337–42.
64. Mellick LB, McIlrath ST, Gellick GA. Treatment of headaches in the ED with lower cervical intramuscular bupivacaine injections: a 1-year retrospective review of 417 patients. Headache. 2006;46:1441–9.
65. Friedman BW, Bijur PE, Lipton RB. Standardizing emergency department-based migraine research: an analysis of commonly used clinical trial outcome measures. Acad Emerg Med. 2010;17:72–9.
66. Friedman BW, Solorzano C, Esses D, et al. Treating headache recurrence after emergency department discharge: a randomized controlled trial of naproxen versus sumatriptan. Ann Emerg Med. 2010;56(1):7–17.
67. Rowe BH, Colman I, Edmonds ML, et al. Randomized controlled trial of intravenous dexamethasone to prevent relapse in acute migraine headaches. Headache. 2008;48:3330340.
68. Fiesseler FW, Shih R, Szucs P, et al. Steroids for migraine headaches: a randomized double-blind, two-armed, placebo-controlled trial. J Emerg Med. 2011;40(4):463–8.
69. Singh A, Alter HJ, Zaia B. Does the addition of dexamethasone to standard therapy for acute migraine decrease the incidence of recurrent headache for patients treated in the emergency department? A meta-analysis and systematic review of the literature. Acad Emerg Med. 2008;15:1223–33.
70. Aurora S, Kori S, Barrodale P, Nelsen A, McDonald S. Gastric stasis occurs in spontaneous, visually induced, and interictal migraine. Headache. 2007;47:1443–6.

Chapter 5
Treating the Child and Adolescent with Acute Headache

Key Chapter Points

- The most common acute pediatric headache in the ED is headache related to acute infection.
- Migraine occurs in about one in three children with acute migraine in the ED.
- Children are less able to describe their headaches than adults.
- Both historical and clinical characteristics help identify pediatric patients with probable secondary headache.
- Occipital headache is a red flag in pediatric patients, warranting additional evaluation.

Keywords Anti-emetic • Occipital headache • Respiratory infection • School

Infection is the most common cause of acute pediatric headache in the emergency department (ED). A survey of consecutive pediatric headache patients (ages 2–18) visiting a single ED over a 1-year period included 432 children and adolescents with a mean age of 8.9 years, with 66% of children between ages 6 and 12 [1]. Over 90% of cases had been experiencing headache for <2 months prior to the visit. Common specific diagnoses were infections of the sinuses, ears, adenoids, or respiratory tract (31%) (see Fig. 5.1 and Table 5.1). Serious intracranial pathology was uncommon.

> *Pearl for the practitioner:*
> The most common diagnosis in pediatric patients presenting to the ED with headache is secondary headache due to infection. Migraine is diagnosed in about 30% of patients. Serious intracranial pathology is identified in <10%.

D.A. Marcus and P.A. Bain, *Practical Assessment and Treatment of the Patient with Headaches in the Emergency Department and Urgent Care Clinic*, DOI 10.1007/978-1-4614-0002-8_5, © Springer Science+Business Media, LLC 2011

Parents are often concerned that pediatric headache is caused by a brain tumor. Fortunately, brain tumors are an infrequent cause of pediatric headache. Similar to adult headache, headache characteristics are generally nonspecific for pediatric patients. Also, as in adults, pediatric headache rarely occurs as an isolated symptom of brain tumor. The Childhood Brain Tumor Consortium is comprised of ten hospitals

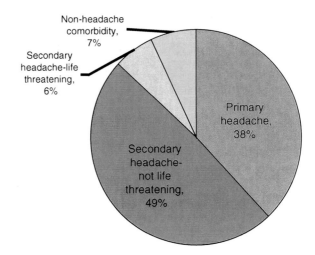

Fig. 5.1 Etiology of acute pediatric headache in the ED (based on [1]). Nonheadache comorbidity describes children presenting with headache but discharged with a diagnosis not demonstrated to be causally related to the headache, including epilepsy, vertigo, syncope, and urticaria. Headache occurring within 3 h of a seizure and resolving within 72 h (called *postictal headache*) occurs commonly in young adults with epilepsy, especially after generalized tonic–clonic seizures [17]

Table 5.1 Specific etiologies of consecutive pediatric patients seen in the ED for headache (based on [1])

General diagnostic category					
Primary headache		**Secondary headache**			
38% of all patients		Not-life threatening 49% of all patients		Life threatening 6% of all patients	
Diagnosis	Percent	Diagnosis	Percent	Diagnosis	Percent
Migraine	29	ENT ID	17	Viral meningitis	2
Tension-type	7	Respiratory ID	14	VP shunt failure	1
Chronic HA	1	Post-trauma HA	9	Brain tumor	1
Cluster HA	1	Drug effect	2	Brain malformation	1
Migraine-related seizure	1	Vision problem	2	Benign intracranial hypertension	1
		Viral ID	1		
		Hypertension	1		
		Dehydration	1		
		Postcraniotomy	1		
		Tooth disorder	1		
		Anemia	<1		

ENT ID sinusitis, otitis, adenoiditis, *HA* headache, *ID* infectious disease, *VP* ventriculo-peritoneal

in the USA and Canada. Data from those patients in the Childhood Brain Tumor Consortium database with headache and brain tumor ($N = 2{,}031$) showed that, similar to adult patients, headache almost always occurred with other troublesome symptoms, with over 99% of children with brain tumors reporting at least one other symptom and over two-thirds reporting at least three other symptoms (Table 5.2) [2]. Furthermore, 98% of children with a headache caused by brain tumor had an abnormal neurological examination. Over half of children with a headache caused by brain tumor had at least five neurological signs (57% of patients with supratentorial tumor and 71% with infratentorial tumor) (see Table 5.3). While these data did not specifically evaluate children seen the ED for headache and brain tumor, they do support that headache will rarely be an isolated or predominant symptom or sign in children with pediatric brain tumor.

Table 5.2 Symptoms typically experienced by children with pediatric brain tumor with headache (based on [2])

Additional nonheadache symptoms in children with headache and brain tumor			
Supratentorial tumors with headache		Intratentorial tumors with headache	
Symptom	Percent	Symptom	Percent
Visual problems other than diplopia	90	Difficulty walking	92
Pain in the back or abdomen	90	Nausea/vomiting	86
Change in academic performance, personality, or speech	87	Pain in the back or abdomen	84
Upper extremity weakness	79	Visual problems other than diplopia	82
Difficulty walking	77	Change in academic performance, personality, or speech	81
Nausea/vomiting	72	Weight loss	79

Table 5.3 Neurological signs that typically present in children with pediatric brain tumor with headache that would be identified on a 5-min neuro screening exam [Chap. 2] (based on [2])

Neurological signs in children with headache and brain tumor			
Supratentorial tumors with headache		Intratentorial tumors with headache	
Sign	Percent	Sign	Percent
Lethargy	71	Gait ataxia	90
Papilledema	65	Uncoordinated limb movements	83
Decreased deep tendon reflexes	56	Papilledema	81
Uncoordinated limb movements	45	Lethargy	77
Up going toe on Babinski	43	Nystagmus[a]	64
Facial weakness	34	Decreased deep tendon reflexes	58
Gait ataxia	31	Sixth nerve palsy[b]	35
Extremity weakness	31	Up going toe on Babinski	35

[a] Rapid, rhythmic, oscillating eye movements
[b] One eye unable to look to the side

> **Pearl for the practitioner:**
> Headache is rarely an isolated symptom in children with brain tumor. Most children with brain tumor report additional symptoms and have an abnormal neurological screening examination.

Although headache descriptions are generally nonspecific in patients with headache due to brain tumor, children with occipital headache should receive additional evaluations to rule out secondary causes of headache, like mass lesions. In one emergency department study, 150 consecutive children presenting to the ED with abrupt onset, severe headaches were prospectively evaluated. In this study, the only two children reporting occipital pain were both diagnosed with posterior fossa tumors [3]. Children and adolescents with occipital headache should receive additional evaluation (e.g., neuroimaging) for possible secondary headaches, even when other symptoms and signs are absent. The combination of occipital headache, neck pain, and neck hyperextension suggests possible brain herniation and requires immediate neurosurgical evaluation [4].

> **Pearl for the practitioner:**
> Occipital headache is a red flag for children in the ED with headache.

Assessment

As with adults, the evaluation of pediatric patients presenting with acute headache begins with a thorough history, using those principles described in Chap. 2 (Table 5.4). History taking can be more challenging from younger patients, who have had less experience evaluating and describing symptoms. As is often seen with pediatric headache, children evaluated in the survey described above had difficulty providing headache descriptions [1]. In this survey, only 28% could describe a pain location and only 8% a pain quality. All but 13 children rated their headache as severe.

Table 5.4 Common pediatric headache conditions based on responses to six essential questions (Chap. 2)

New headache	Problem with chronic headache	Headache PLUS something else	Headache in patient with known illness
Infection	Migraine	Carbon monoxide poisoning or other exposure	Ventriculo-peritoneal shunt failure
Trauma			
Substance abuse		Tumor	
Hemorrhage			

Secondary Headaches

Historical and physical examination features can be used to distinguish probable primary from probable secondary headaches (Table 5.5). Imaging studies are generally best reserved for patients with traumatic headache, a known neurological condition (e.g., ventriculo-peritoneal shunt even when infection is absent), or neurological signs/symptoms [5]. Routinely imaging headache patients may lead to false diagnoses, as illustrated by the cases.

Pearl for the practitioner:
Neuroimaging for pediatric headache is usually reserved for cases with

- Trauma
- Known neurological disorder (e.g., prior brain surgery)
- Neurological symptoms (e.g., seizure, confusion, focal deficits)
- Neurological signs (e.g., papilledema, mental status changes, focal deficits)

Case

Two adolescents presenting to the ED with new onset, nontraumatic headache were evaluated with magnetic imaging studies, both of which were interpreted as Chiari malformation (images A and B). Patient A reported new onset monthly frontal headaches starting 3 months after menarche and associated with blurred vision, dizziness, and marked nausea during the headache episodes. Between episodes, she remained symptom free and her general medical and neurological examinations are normal. Although she has symptoms of dizziness, blurred vision, and nausea, which may occur in symptomatic Chiari patients, these symptoms are isolated to her headache episodes. She is appropriately diagnosed with migraine. Patient B likewise reports new onset headaches. She reports headaches starting at the back of the head and neck that are markedly aggravated by coughing or straining to have a bowel movement. Her mother also reports that she has gagged on food several times during the last few months, which has never happened before. Although she has always considered herself to be fairly athletic and coordinated, over the last several months she reports feeling "off-balance" and has had several minor injuries in gym class from falling or getting hit with balls that she was too slow to avoid. Her examination reveals abnormal eye movements and scoliosis. Her headaches and other neurological symptoms may be attributed to the Chiari malformation.

(continued)

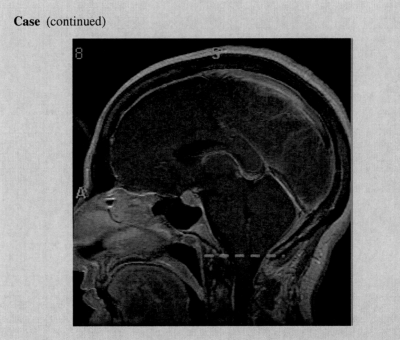

Image A. Only about 1 mm of cerebellar tissue dips below the yellow line, representing the location of the foramen magnum, in this patient with an asymptomatic Chiari Type I malformation (photo courtesy of Rock Heyman, MD)

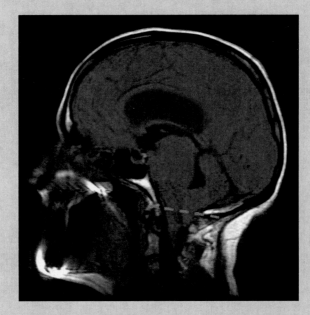

Image B. Substantial cerebellar and brainstem tissue dips below the foramen magnum in this patient with a symptomatic Chiari Type II malformation (photo courtesy of Rock Heyman, MD)

(continued)

Case (continued)

A Chiari malformation may be diagnosed when cerebellar tissue passes into the foramen magnum. A Type I malformation involves an extension of the cerebellar tonsils only (Image A) and is often an incidental, asymptomatic finding. Type II involves extension of both cerebellum and brainstem tissue through the foramen magnum (Image B), which may produce symptoms of head and neck pain, dizziness or balance problems, vision problems, motor deficits, etc. Chiari malformations may also be associated with spina bifida, syringomyelia, and other neurological conditions. Interestingly, although a Chiari malformation is congenital and present at birth, symptoms are often delayed until later childhood, adolescence, or early adulthood. Symptoms may occur with Type I Chiari as well as more severe types, although headache usually does not occur in isolation. Patients with symptomatic Chiari malformation will usually report a variety of symptoms:

- Headache and neck pain, with pain usually at the base of the skull and worsened with Valsalva maneuvers, coughing, or sneezing
- Coordination or balance problems or unsteady gait
- Tingling and numbness in the extremities
- Swallowing problems, including problems with choking
- Blurred or double vision
- Slurred speech

Table 5.5 Clues that pediatric ED headache may be a secondary headache (based on [1])

	Primary headache	Secondary headache
Pain location	Unilateral pain	Poorly localized or occipital pain
Pain quality	Pulsing or constrictive	Unable to describe
Pain severity	Severe	Slight or very intense
Associated symptoms	Photophobia, phonophobia	Fever, focal neurological deficits, behavioral disturbances
Associated signs	None	Papilledema, ataxia, hemiparesis, abnormal eye movements

Vomiting did not distinguish primary from secondary headache, occurring in 30% of patients with either type of headache

Table 5.6 Diagnostic distinctions between pediatric and adult migraine (based on [6])

	Adult	Pediatric
Location	Unilateral	Often bilateral. Occipital migraine is rare and warrants additional evaluation
Duration	4–72 h	1–72 h
Associated symptoms	Photophobia and phonophobia are usually present	Children rarely verbalize sensitivity to noise and lights; photo- and phono-phobia may be inferred from behavior (e.g., retreating to dark, quiet room; turning off television or computer)

Migraine

Children with migraine often lack features characteristic of adult migraine (Table 5.6) [6]. Compared with adult migraine, pediatric migraine is more likely to be

- Bilateral;
- Diffuse and frontotemporal in location;
- Shorter in duration (often <2 h);
- Without associated photophobia and phonophobia reported.

Occipital headaches are unusual in children and should warrant consideration of a more extensive work-up.

> **Pearl for the practitioner:**
> Pediatric ED patients describing a unilateral headache are more likely to have a primary headache than a secondary headache condition [1]. In most cases, children with migraine describe their headache as bilateral or diffuse.

Treatment

Among patients with secondary headaches, headache management is generally symptomatic with the primary treatment focused on the causative condition.

Pediatric and Adolescent Migraine in the ED

Similar to adult migraine, most ED doctors treat pediatric migraine with anti-emetics and analgesics. A retrospective survey evaluated treatment given to 1,694 pediatric patients seen in the ED for migraine (mean age = 12.1 years) [7]. Migraine attacks had lasted for an average of 2.2 days prior to the ED visit. Before coming to the ED,

63% of patients had used some migraine treatment, most commonly acetaminophen, ibuprofen, or other oral analgesic (53%), with 5% having used an opioid and 2% a triptan. In the ED, most patients were treated with a dopamine antagonist (metoclopramide, prochlorperazine, or chlorpromazine) or oral analgesic (acetaminophen or ibuprofen) (see Fig. 5.2). Dihydroergotamine (DHE) and triptans were used, respectively, by only 0.9% and 0.5% of patients.

Focusing treatment on anti-emetics and analgesics is supported by a summary of efficacy for childhood and adolescent headache treatment based on 14 randomized, controlled clinical trials (Table 5.7) [8]. Only one study was performed in the ED, however, which limits the usefulness of these results for evaluating ED treatment. Overall, the more effective treatments for reducing migraine pain included analgesics and prochlorperazine. None of the treatments consistently resulted in a pain-free response nor were any consistently beneficial for preventing headache recurrence or the need to use additional rescue medications.

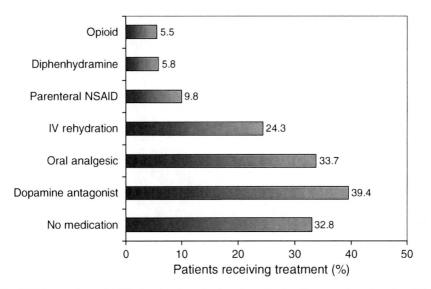

Fig. 5.2 Commonly used (≥5% of patients) medications for pediatric migraine patients (based on [7])

Table 5.7 Comparison of controlled trials evaluating pediatric acute migraine treatments (based on [8])

Route of delivery and medication tested	Benefit for pain relief
Oral agents	
Acetaminophen	Effective
Ibuprofen	Effective
Triptans	Inconsistent results
DHE	Ineffective
Intranasal agents	
Sumatriptan	Inconsistent results
Intravenous agents	
Prochlorperazine	Effective; more effective than ketorolac

In a retrospective survey of 92 pediatric patients treated in the ED with intravenous prochlorperazine with diphenhydramine for severe migraine, treatment failure (defined as need for additional rescue therapy, hospitalization, or return to the ED within 48 h for headache recurrence or medication side effect) occurred in 14% [9]. Eight patients required additional therapy and five patients (including three for whom additional therapy was used) were hospitalized. Among those discharged, three returned for headache recurrence.

Triptans have shown inconsistent benefit in studies testing children and adolescents (Table 5.7), however, they are often useful when nonopioid analgesics either at home or in the ED have been ineffective.

Dosing Migraine Treatments for Children and Adolescents

The same treatments used for adult headache are often effective in pediatric patients, although dosage adjustment will be necessary. The European Federation of Neurological Sciences task force provided guidelines for effective acute migraine treatment in children and adolescents (Table 5.8) [10]. These same recommendations were echoed in a subsequent report by the European Headache Federation [11, 12]. When these medications are ineffective or nausea is pronounced and additional anti-emetic therapy is needed, additional medications recommended in Chap. 4 may also be tried as second-line therapy, using pediatric dosing based on age and weight.

Anesthetic Therapy

Bilateral lower cervical paraspinous intramuscular bupivacaine injections were shown to be effective headache treatment in a small retrospective study of 13 pediatric headache patients who had experienced headache for an average of 3.2 days before coming to the ED [13]. Complete relief of headache occurred in six patients, with partial relief in five patients.

Discharge Information

Parent education about migraine and appropriate lifestyle modifications is essential, especially for parents with children or adolescents experiencing frequent disabling

Table 5.8 Effective acute migraine drugs in children and adolescents (based on [10]; rizatriptan dosing based on [12])

Treatment	Dosage
Ibuprofen	10 mg/kg
Acetaminophen/paracetamol	15 mg/kg
Domperidone (for nausea)	10 mg (not available in Canada and the USA)
Sumatriptan nasal spray	10 mg after age 12
Zolmitriptan	5 mg nasal spray or 2.5–5 mg oral after age 12
Rizatriptan	5 mg for children weighing 20–39 kg and 10 mg for children ≥40 kg

> **Box 5.1** ED Headache Treatment Options for Pediatric Patients
>
> - Ice pack, massage, neck stretches
> - Reduced lights, reduced noise, soothing music
> - Intravenous rehydration
> - Anti-emetic
>   - Prochlorperazine (Compazine) 0.1–0.15 mg/kg PO, IM, or IV (maximum dose 10 mg). Pre-treat with diphenhydramine 1–2 mg/kg
>   - Ondansetron (Zofran) 0.15 mg/kg PO, IM, or IV (children weighing >40 kg are usually treated with a single 4 mg dose; maximum dose 8 mg)
>   - Metoclopramide (Reglan) 0.1–0.2 mg/kg IM or IV (maximum dose 10 mg). Pretreat with diphenhydramine 1–2 mg/kg
> - Analgesic
>   - Ketorolac (Toradol) 0.5–1.0 mg/kg (maximum dose 30 mg IM, 15 mg IV)
>   - Sumatriptan (Imitrex) 3 mg SQ (may use 6 mg SQ in patients >30 kg).
> - Consider trigger point injections or nerve blocks in select patients
>
> IM = intramuscular; IV = intravenous; PO = oral; SQ = subcutaneous

attacks [14]. While migraine education will occur in detail during appropriate outpatient follow-up, the ED staff can begin this important process by providing written information to help reinforce healthy lifestyle habits essential for long-term headache management in children and adolescents (Box 5.2). This information can help answer questions about activity level and school attendance that many parents will have before leaving the ED. Children and adolescents respond well to relaxation techniques [15, 16] and instruction sheets on relaxation (Chap. 4) should also be provided at discharge.

Additional Resources for Treating Pediatric Headache

- *Pediatric Migraine Headache: An Evidenced-Based Approach (Pediatric Emergency Medicine Practice)* by Cole S. Condra and Jane F. Knapp, 2010.
- *Pediatric Headaches in Clinical Practice* by Andrew D. Hershey, Scott W. Powers, Paul Winner, and Marielle A. Kabbouche, 2009.
- *Headache and your Child: The Complete Guide to Understanding and Treating Migraine and Other Headaches in Children and Adolescents* by Seymour Diamond and Amy Diamond, 2001.
- *Headache in Children and Adolescents* by Paul Winner and A. David Rothner, 2001.

Box 5.2 Parent instructions for dealing with a child or adolescent with migraine (based on [14]).

Migraine is a recurring headache condition that often runs in families. If your child has migraines, it is likely that one of his parents or other relatives also get migraine headaches. People with migraines will usually have headaches every few days or weeks. For this reason, it is essential that you talk to your child's doctor about what to do to help prevent and treat future headaches that are likely to occur.

What Can My Child Take When He or She Gets a Migraine?

Talk to your doctor to find out the best medication treatment for your young person. Over-the-counter analgesics and prescription migraine drugs usually help. Specific recommendations will depend on what your youth's headaches are like and how often they occur.

- Taking analgesics too often can worsen migraines, so make sure you talk to your doctor about what to give your child and how often it can be used
- Never give your child your migraine medications. Although many of the same drugs can be used for both children and adults with migraines, doses are usually different. In addition, having other health problems or concerns about side effects will often affect the drugs your doctor will recommend you can safely use in your child or adolescent
- Give medications and instructions on how medications are to be used to the school nurse to have on hand for migraines that happen during the school day

What Can I Do to Help Reduce My Child's Headaches?

First, let your child or adolescent know that the headaches are caused by migraine, that they will likely come back every so often, but that there are many things they can do to make the headaches less of a problem.

Structure Your Child's Schedule

Migraines often occur when there has been a break in the regular routine or new stresses. Trying to keep your child on a regular routine can help reduce how often migraines occur.

- *Make sure your child's getting enough sleep.* Children and adolescents need more sleep than adults. Typical sleep requirements depend on your youngster's age:
  - Toddlers need to sleep 10–12 h at night
  - Elementary students need 10 h of sleep

- Teenagers still need more than 9 h of sleep each night
- If your child or adolescent cannot fit in all of his or her after-school activities, dinner, homework, and adequate sleep time, reduce the amount of after-school commitments

- *Keep a regular bedtime.* Bedtime needs to be no later than 10 p.m. If your child or adolescent is unable to sleep, she can be allowed to listen to the radio or read a book. She should not be watching television, texting, talking on the telephone, or snacking after bedtime
- *Set a regular time to get up.* This time needs to allow adequate time for getting ready for school. Regular bed and rise times need to be maintained even for kids who are already out of school on homebound education
- *Maintain regular meal times.* Your adolescent must eat breakfast, lunch, and dinner everyday. Skipping meals is a common headache trigger
- *Maintain a regular homework.* Schedule a regular homework time and location that's not in front of the television or computer games
- *Maintain enjoyable leisure activities.* These activities will preferably take your child out of the house and encourage socialization. Limit time playing computer games or surfing the Internet. Limit time spent watching television or movies. Encourage activities like walking, shopping, sports, and socializing

Identify Stress Factors in Your Youngster's Life

Stress is the most common migraine trigger for both children and adults. There are many circumstances that increase stress for children and adolescents. These may include

- School course work
- Difficulty interacting with a peer group or bullying
- Excessive after school commitments
- Depression
- Anxiety
- Fears of health conditions or illness
- Family strife
- Sexual issues
- Drug exposure or pressure

These should be addressed by your child's doctor, psychologist, or counselor.

What About School?

Research shows that most youngsters have their migraines on school days during regular school hours. This does not mean they are faking the headaches to get out of school. School can be very stressful for young people – for academic, athletic, and social reasons. Missing school, however, adds extra stress that can further aggravate headaches.

Good school participation, including regular attendance, must be a top priority. In most cases, your child should attend school – even when she has a migraine.

- Migraines usually go away after 1 or 2 h, so your child shouldn't need to miss a day of school for a migraine
- Going to school usually won't make a headache any worse. In fact, being at school can help distract your child from headache symptoms
- If your child gets frequent headaches, he should probably only miss school time when vomiting and should attend school later that day once the headache symptoms lessen

Talk to your youngster's teacher and nurse to let them know that your young person has migraines and what has been recommended for treatment. If headaches occur during the school day, the child should be allowed to leave the classroom to go to the nurse. The nurse may administer prescribed medication and allow the child to use pain management techniques, like relaxation techniques. Unless the child is vomiting, he or she should return to the classroom after 15–20 min.

School is important for social, emotional, and intellectual development. If a child or adolescent has been unable to attend school, work with your youngster's healthcare provider, school nurses, guidance counselors, and teachers to help make a successful return to school and then to maintain attendance. A return to school can begin with attending low-stress classes and lunch period.

Summary

- About 60% of pediatric ED headaches will be caused by a secondary headache.
- Children presenting to the ED for headache most commonly have an infectious diagnosis of the sinuses, ears, adenoids, or respiratory tract.
- Pediatric patients will require additional testing to rule out secondary headaches when their pain is occipital or fever, neurological signs or symptoms, or behavioral changes are present. Doctors should also be suspicious of mild severity headaches that bring patients to the ED.
- Similar to adults, pediatric migraine in the ED is usually best treated with anti-emetics, analgesics, and intravenous hydration.
- Dosage adjustments are usually needed, based on age and weight.
- Nondrug treatments should be encouraged and reinforced with written instructions.

References

1. Conicella E, Raucci U, Vanacore N, et al. The child with headache in a pediatric emergency department. Headache. 2008;48:1005–11.
2. The Childhood Brain Tumor Consortium. The epidemiology of headache among children with brain tumor. Headache in children with brain tumors. J Neurooncol. 1991;10:31–46.
3. Lewis DW, Qureshi F. Acute headache in children and adolescents presenting to the emergency department. Headache. 2000;40:200–3.
4. Nazemi KJ, Malempati S. Emergency department presentation of childhood cancer. Emerg Med Clin N Am. 2009;27:477–95.
5. Kan L, Nagelberg J, Maytal J. Headaches in a pediatric emergency department: etiology, imaging, and treatment. Headache. 2000;40:25–9.
6. Headache Classification Committee of the International Headache Society. The international classification of headache disorders, 2nd edition. Cephalalgia. 2004;24 Suppl 1:24–5.
7. Richer LP, Laycock K, Millar K, et al. Treatment of children with migraine in emergency departments: national practice variation study. Pediatrics. 2010;126:e150–5.
8. Bailey B, McManus BC. Treatment of children with migraine in the emergency department. A qualitative systematic review. Ped Emerg Care. 2008;24:321–30.
9. Trottier ED, Bailey B, Dauphin-Pierre S, Gravel J. Clinical outcomes of children treated with intravenous prochlorperazine for migraine in a pediatric emergency department. J Emerg Med. 2010;39:166–73.
10. Evers A, Áfra J, Frese A, et al. EFNS guideline on the drug treatment of migraine – revised report of an EFNS task force. Eur J Neurol. 2009;16(9):968–81.
11. Steiner TJ, Paemeleire K, Jensen R, et al. European principles of management of common headache disorders in primary care. J Headache Pain. 2007;8:S3–21.
12. Ahonen K, Hämäläinen ML, Eerola M, Hoppu K. A randomized trial of rizatriptan in migraine attacks in children. Neurology. 2006;67:1135–40.
13. Mellick LB, Pleasant MR. Do pediatric headaches respond to bilateral lower cervical paraspinous bupivacaine injections? Pediatr Emerg Care. 2010;26:192–6.
14. Marcus DA. Reducing headache disability in children and adolescents. Am Fam Physician. 2002;65:554–8.
15. Sartory G, Muller B, Metsch J, Pothmann R. A comparison of psychological and pharmacological treatment of pediatric migraine. Behav Res Ther. 1998;36:1155–70.
16. Scharff L, Marcus D, Masek BJ. A controlled study of minimal-contact thermal biofeedback in children with migraine. J Pediatr Psychol. 2002;27:109–19.
17. Ekstein D, Schachter SS. Postictal headache. Epilepsy Behav. 2010;19:151–5.

Chapter 6
Treatment of Pregnant and Breastfeeding Patients with Acute Headache in the ED

Key Chapter Points

- Most headaches occurring during pregnancy and breastfeeding are benign, primary headaches.
- Secondary headaches should be ruled out in pregnant and nursing women using necessary testing, including spinal fluid examination and neuroimaging, when appropriate.
- The anti-emetic of choice for pregnant and lactating women is ondansetron.
- Pain medication treatments of choice for pregnant women include intravenous therapy with ketorolac (second trimester only), magnesium, or hydromorphone. Intranasal lidocaine drops are safe and sometimes helpful for migraine.
- Pain medication treatments of choice for lactating women include subcutaneous sumatriptan or intravenous therapy with ketorolac, valproate (provided that reliable contraception can be ensured), magnesium, or hydromorphone. Ketorolac may also be given intramuscularly. Prochlorperazine can be used to help relieve both nausea and other migraine symptoms during lactation.
- Patients with residual headache after standard treatments may benefit from trigger point injections, a greater occipital nerve block, or a short course of prednisone.

Keywords Breastfeeding • Conception • Dehydration • Lactation • Nursing • Pregnancy

Headache is one of the most common physical complaints reported during pregnancy. In one survey of women attending a university obstetric clinic, common physical complaints in pregnant women identified through a standard questionnaire included back pain (81%), nausea (72%), extremity or joint pain (59%), stomach pain (57%), digestive problems (50%), shortness of breath (49%), and headaches (49%) [1]. Headaches occurring during pregnancy and postpartum are usually

D.A. Marcus and P.A. Bain, *Practical Assessment and Treatment of the Patient* 133
with Headaches in the Emergency Department and Urgent Care Clinic,
DOI 10.1007/978-1-4614-0002-8_6, © Springer Science+Business Media, LLC 2011

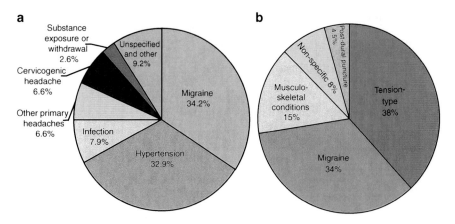

Fig. 6.1 Headache diagnoses during pregnancy and after delivery. (**a**) Prospective evaluation of new onset headache during pregnancy (based on [2]). (**b**) Postpartum headache diagnoses (based on [3])

Box 6.1 Common Secondary Causes of Headache During Pregnancy

- Dehydration
- Infection
- Preeclampsia/eclampsia
- Trauma
- Acute stroke
- Vascular events

  - Ruptured arteriovenous malformations or cerebral aneurysms
  - Stroke
  - Cervicocranial dissection
  - Postpartum cerebral venous thrombosis (usually during the first 2 weeks postpartum) [52]

- Increased intracranial pressure

  - Brain tumor (pituitary adenoma and meningioma growth are accelerated during pregnancy [53, 54])
  - Idiopathic intracranial hypertension (may also be triggered by elevated estrogen, and may occur or worsen during pregnancy [55–58])

---

caused by benign, primary headaches, especially migraine and tension-type (Fig. 6.1) [2, 3]. Secondary headaches, however, also need to be considered (Box 6.1).

Secondary headaches related to pregnancy include cerebral venous thrombosis (Table 6.1 and Fig. 6.2) and eclampsia/preeclampsia (Table 6.2 and Case). Eclampsia is diagnosed when a patient with preeclampsia develops new onset generalized seizures or unexplained loss of consciousness. In one survey, 38% of patients with eclampsia had seizures before hypertension and proteinuria had been documented [4]. Most cases of eclampsia occur during the third trimester or within the first 2 days after delivery.

Table 6.1 Symptoms in
women with cerebral venous
and sinus thrombosis
($N=465$; 77 women were
pregnant or postpartum) [60]

Symptoms, signs, and findings	Percentage
Symptom	
Headache	91
Seizure	39
Paresis	37
Mental status change	20
Aphasia	19
Sensory symptoms	6
Signs/findings	
Intracranial hemorrhage or infarct	65
Papilledema	28
Coma	5

Pearl for the practitioner:
Most headaches encountered in pregnant patients are benign. Secondary headaches (e.g., headaches caused by infections, preeclampsia/eclampsia, vascular disease, and increased intracranial pressure) are much less common, but should be kept in mind when assessing a pregnant woman with headaches.

Case

Sarah is a 27-year-old primigravida with a history of menstrual migraine since starting her menstrual periods at age 13. She is currently at gestational week 24 of an uncomplicated pregnancy. Sarah has been nearly headache-free since beginning her second trimester and presents to the ED with a complaint of throbbing headache that is more severe than her typical menstrual migraine and associated with blurred vision, photophobia, and seeing spots, although she has never had an aura with her migraines. She has also noticed swelling in her hands so that she stopped wearing rings. She additionally reports pain under her ribs on the right side. Hypertension (145/92 mmHg) and proteinuria confirm the diagnosis of preeclampsia.

Sarah's case highlights the need to consider possible secondary headaches, even in young, healthy women with a history of migraine. Interestingly, women with migraine are at higher risk for developing preeclampsia. In a retrospective survey, migraine was significantly more common among women with preeclampsia vs. those without (14% vs. 5%, odds ratio=2.87, $P<0.05$) [51].

Expected Changes in Primary Headaches During Pregnancy and Delivery

Migraine and, to a lesser extent, tension-type headache typically improve during the first trimester of pregnancy. Retrospective studies report spontaneous improvement in 50–80% of pregnant women with migraine and 30% with tension-type headache

Fig. 6.2 Sagittal sinus thrombosis (image courtesy of Clayton A. Wiley, MD). (**a**) Magnetic resonance (MR) arteriography. Special MR imaging techniques allow visualization of the blood vessels of the brain. Here, the bright signal indicates venous drainage from the brain. (**b**) Magnetic resonance imaging, coronal view. In this coronal image of the head, there is abnormal bright signal consistent with superior saggital vein thrombosis above the apex of the brain. Diminished return of blood from the brain will lead to brain swelling, causing severe headache and eventually venous stroke

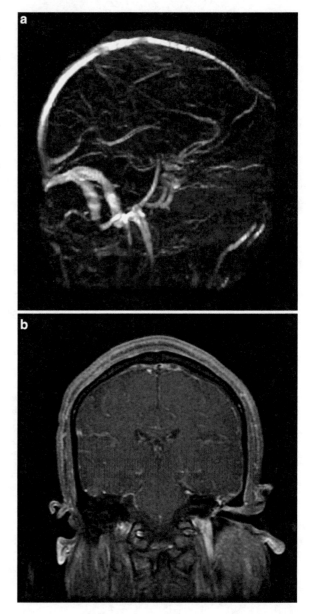

[5–8]. Prospective data likewise support primary headache improvement for most women during pregnancy (Fig. 6.3) [2].

Although most women experience improvement in pre-existing headaches with pregnancy, women reporting ongoing headaches at the end of the first trimester (usually around the time of the first obstetrical visit) are unlikely to experience significant headache improvement during the remainder of pregnancy. A small prospective study of 30 mixed headache sufferers experiencing recurring primary headache at the end of the first trimester showed only an additional 30% improvement between the second and third trimesters, with a slightly greater likelihood of improvement in women with migraine [9]. Even when primary headaches improve with pregnancy, they typically recur soon after delivery (Fig. 6.4) [10].

Table 6.2 Recognizing preeclampsia

Symptoms	Signs/findings
• Severe headache • Light sensitivity, blurred vision, or other visual disturbance • Upper abdominal pain, nausea/vomiting • Dizziness • Weight gain >2 lb in a week • Swelling • Decreased urination	• BP >140/90 in previously normotensive patient; SBP increased ≥30 mmHg or DBP increased ≥15 mmHg in patient with preexisting essential hypertension • Hyperreflexia • Generalized edema • Proteinuria[a] • Abnormal liver function tests • Thrombocytopenia

BP blood pressure, *SBP* systolic blood pressure, *DBP* diastolic blood pressure
[a]Urine dipstick is unreliable. In the ED, a urine protein-to-creatinine ratio ≥0.19 suggests proteinuria [61]

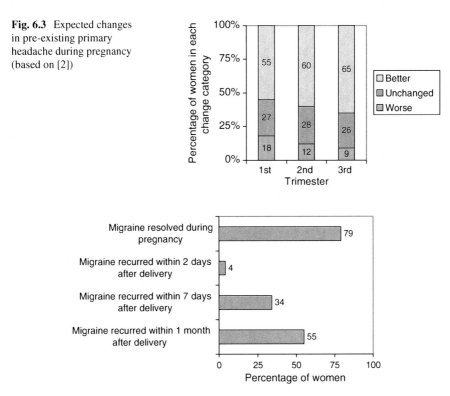

Fig. 6.3 Expected changes in pre-existing primary headache during pregnancy (based on [2])

Fig. 6.4 Headache recurrence after delivery (based on [10]). Breastfeeding offered a protective effect against headache recurrence, with headache recurring within 1 month of delivery in all bottle feeding mothers and only 43% who were breastfeeding

> **Pearl for the practitioner:**
> Migraine improves for at least two in three women during pregnancy. Migraine is expected to recur in most women within a month of delivery.

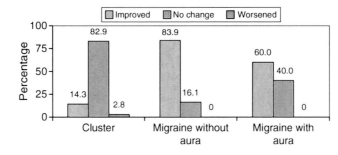

Fig. 6.5 Changes in primary headache during pregnancy (based on [11])

Cluster headache is rarely seen in young women, so this will infrequently be seen in pregnant women. In women with pre-pregnancy cluster headache, the cluster pattern is generally unaffected by pregnancy. In a small study, headache severity during pregnancy was compared in 35 women with cluster headache and 56 women with migraine [11]. Headache generally improved during pregnancy among the women with migraine, with no change among those with cluster headache (Fig. 6.5). A second study of women with cluster headache included 53 women with cluster headache diagnosed before their first pregnancy [12]. Nineteen of these women recalled cluster attacks occurring during pregnancy, with 11 of the 19 women reporting no change in cluster frequency or severity during pregnancy (58%), 3 patients improvement (16%), and 5 patients worsening (26%). Interestingly, women who had started having cluster attacks before they had ever been pregnant were less likely to become pregnant. One-third of those women who chose not to have children cited having cluster headaches as the reason for not pursuing pregnancy.

Testing Women During Pregnancy or While Breastfeeding

The same principles concerning evaluation of headache in nonpregnant patients apply to women during pregnancy and lactation. New headaches or a significant change in headache pattern during pregnancy or after delivery requires a detailed history and physical examination to differentiate benign, primary headaches from pathological headaches. As described in Chaps. 2 and 3, headache associated with papilledema, focal neurological signs or symptoms, or seizures suggests intracranial pathology and necessitates a complete neurological evaluation. Headache associated with trauma or abnormal findings on physical examination (e.g., swelling and hypertension) will also require additional evaluation.

Evaluations that might affect treatment during pregnancy or when nursing should not be delayed until after delivery or discontinuation of nursing. As described in Chap. 3, necessary evaluations typically include a detailed history, physical examination, and any laboratory testing targeted to rule out specific possible secondary headache conditions. Both spinal fluid examinations and radiographic imaging should be included in the evaluation when appropriate and necessary and the results will guide treatment.

Pearl for the practitioner:
Secondary headaches are uncommon in pregnant and breastfeeding women. If secondary headaches are a serious consideration and confirmation of the secondary headache would change therapy, further investigation with spinal fluid analysis and/or imaging procedures should be pursued, as clinically indicated.

Spinal Fluid Assessment

Spinal fluid examinations can be safely performed and easily interpreted in pregnancy, with opening pressure, cell count, and protein levels similar between nonpregnant and pregnant women [13]. Spinal fluid results are unaffected by active labor, length of gestation, and type of delivery (vaginal vs. Cesarean section). Therefore, abnormal values obtained during pregnancy should not be attributed to the pregnancy itself, but must be further evaluated as in the nonpregnant patient.

Radiographic Studies

Plain x-rays are typically avoided during pregnancy, unless treatment during pregnancy will be altered based on results. Patients requiring x-rays should be provided with a pelvic shield to reduce fetal radiation exposure.

Similar to nonpregnant patients, magnetic resonance imaging (MRI) is preferred for pregnant and nursing patients being evaluated for headache. The American College of Radiology recommends MRI during pregnancy to avoid exposure to ionizing radiation when imaging studies are needed and the results of testing may change patient care [14]. MRI exposure during pregnancy is generally considered to be safe [15], with no negative sequelae identified during evaluations of 3-year olds exposed to MRI in utero [16] or the offspring of female MRI technicians [17].

Pearl for the practitioner:
MRI is the preferred neuroimaging study for pregnant and nursing patients being evaluated for headache.

Computed tomography (CT) imaging may be necessary in some women with abnormal neurological examinations or headaches suggesting intracranial hemorrhage. Fetal effects depend on both the timing and dosage of radiation exposure [18]. In general, fetal radiation exposure from a maternal head CT is extremely low (<0.005 mGy), well below levels that have been linked to fetal effects [19–21]. Fetal exposure to ionizing radiation from a maternal head CT is generally considered to be substantially less risky for the fetus than not identifying and treating potentially serious neurological conditions in the mother [22].

> **Pearl for the practitioner:**
> CT testing may be used when medically necessary during pregnancy as fetal radiation exposure from a maternal head CT is generally extremely low.

The 11th European Symposium on Urogenital Radiology conducted an extensive literature review of the use of iodinated and gadolinium contrast during pregnancy and lactation, with a recommendation to use contrast agents when they are deemed necessary during pregnancy and nursing [23]. Iodinated contrast may be used during pregnancy if necessary information will be gathered from the testing. Exposure to maternal iodinated contrast agents can depress fetal and neonatal thyroid function; therefore, exposed newborns should be screened for thyroid function. There are no known human fetal effects from intrauterine gadolinium exposure; however, gadolinium should only be used during pregnancy when the additional information provided by gadolinium contrast is necessary so that benefits outweigh potential risks [24]. Only small amounts of iodinated or gadolinium contrast agents are expected in breast milk; therefore, temporary cessation of breastfeeding is not recommended when either contrast agent is used in lactating women.

> **Pearl for the practitioner:**
> Neuroimaging, including MRI and CT testing with contrast, should not be withheld from patients who are pregnant or nursing if the information that might be obtained from imaging may change treatment.

The importance of not foregoing neuroimaging studies for pregnant patients considered to be candidates for evaluation was highlighted in a retrospective review of 63 pregnant women reporting to an emergency department (ED) for a primary complaint of headache. Those evaluated with magnetic resonance or computed tomography studies had normal studies or only incidental/nonspecific findings in 73% of women; a pathological condition was identified in 27% (Fig. 6.6) [25]. Among patients with abnormal neurological examinations, a pathological brain

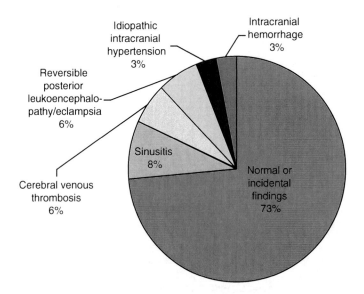

Fig. 6.6 Neuroimaging abnormalities identified in pregnant patients seen in the ED for headache and sent for a magnetic resonance or computed tomography scan (based on [25])

scan was identified in 38% of patients; while 19% with a normal neurological examination had a pathological brain scan. This study highlights several important points about neuroimaging during pregnancy:

1. Important pathological conditions may occur in women seeking ED treatment for headache and these conditions can be confirmed with neuroimaging.
2. Patients for whom evaluation suggests a possible secondary headache should not be restricted from neuroimaging due to pregnancy, even when their neurological examination is normal.

Treatment During Pregnancy and Lactation

Safety Rating Systems

ED medication treatment during pregnancy and breastfeeding generally utilizes more limited drug choices to maximize safety for the baby. Drug safety during pregnancy has been categorized using several systems, including the Food and Drug Administration System (FDA), the Teratogen Information System (TERIS), and numerous systems in Europe. TERIS rates risk of teratogenic effects for the offspring of exposed women as none, minimal, small, moderate, or high. Agreement among these systems for the safety of individual drugs is fairly poor [26]. The most commonly used system in the USA is the FDA rating, which is currently under

Box 6.2 Proposed Revisions to the FDA Pregnancy Rating System

Old FDA risk-category rating		Proposed updated FDA descriptions
Category	Definition	
A	*Safety has been established* through controlled studies	• Fetal risk summary, including risk for malformation, mortality, and growth retardation
B	*Safety is likely* based on safety shown in animal studies with no controlled human studies OR adverse events were seen in animal studies but not confirmed in controlled human studies	
C	*Teratogenicity is possible* based on adverse events in animal studies with no controlled human studies OR neither animal nor human studies are available. Most drugs are in this category due to lack of available data	• Clinical considerations during pregnancy and lactation, including consequences of inadvertent exposures • Prescribing information, including timing during pregnancy
D	*Teratogenicity is probable* based on human studies; however, benefits may be acceptable despite possible risk (e.g., drug is needed in a life-threatening situation or for a serious disease for which safer drugs cannot be used or are ineffective)	• Data section providing detailed discussion of known information
X	*Teratogenicity is likely* and the drug is contraindicated in pregnancy	

revision (Box 6.2). Rather than providing sequential rankings, the new system will provide descriptive data, detailing known information for each drug.

Rehydration

Adequate hydration is particularly important for pregnant and lactating women. Maternal dehydration affects fetal amniotic fluid dynamics and may contribute to the development of oligohydramnios (i.e., decreased amniotic fluid volume) [27]. Although dehydration has been anecdotally linked to increased risk for preterm labor, benefits from hydration for preventing preterm labor are inconsistent [28]. Dehydration also increases risks for developing thrombotic disorders, such as stroke, presumably due to increased viscosity [29].

Rehydration during pregnancy should occur with intravenous fluids. While specific data on the effects of rehydration in pregnant women are lacking, an interesting study using pregnant sheep detailed effects on both the sheep and fetal lamb from rehydration after dehydration using oral or intravenous maternal rehydration [30]. Arterial and urinary chemistry and hormonal levels, as well as cardiovascular markers, were assessed. Although maternal recovery occurred with either oral or intravenous rehydration, positive changes were seen early in the fetus only with maternal intravenous rehydration. While similar studies evaluating rehydration in humans are not available, animal data may support using intravenous dehydration as standard rehydration treatment during pregnancy.

Treating Migraine During Pregnancy

Preferred medications for migraine in women who are pregnant are described in Table 6.3. A checklist describing typical migraine treatment options for pregnant women is provided in Box 6.3.

Table 6.3 Preferred ED headache treatment during pregnancy

First choice	Second choice	Other
Nonmedication therapies	Magnesium sulfate	Occipital nerve blocks
Rehydration	Tramadol (Ultram)	Trigger point injections
Ondansetron (Zofran)		Lidocaine nasal spray
Ketorolac (Toradol) – second trimester only		Hydromorphone (Dilaudid) as rescue therapy

Box 6.3 ED Headache Treatment Options During Pregnancy (Adapted from Marcus DA, Bain PA. Effective migraine treatment in pregnant and lactating women. New York: Springer; 2009)

- Urgent care/ED treatments
    - Ice pack, massage, neck stretches
    - Reduced lights, reduced noise, soothing music
    - Intravenous rehydration
    - Anti-emetic
        - IV ondansetron (Zofran) 4–8 mg over 2–5 min (preferred)
        - IM promethazine (Phenergan) 12.5–25 mg, with monitoring for akathisia
        - IV/IM prochlorperazine (Compazine) 5–10 mg (over 5 min if IV), with monitoring for akathisia
    - Analgesic
        - Hydromorphone (Dilaudid) 1–2 mg IM/SQ or 0.5–1 mg IV over 2–3 min
    - Anesthetic
        - Occipital nerve blocks
        - Trigger point injections
        - Intranasal 4% lidocaine (needs to be compounded) 10–20 drops (0.5–1 mL) into nostril on side of the headache while lying on the back with neck extended; may be repeated in 2 min, if needed

(continued)

Box 6.3 (continued)

- Discharge medication recommendations
  - Anti-emetic
    - Ondansetron 4–8 mg 1/2–1 tablet every 6 h as needed for severe nausea (patients may prefer orally dissolvable tablet)
    - Prochlorperazine 10 mg PO every 6 h as needed
    - Prochlorperazine 25 mg PR every 6 h as needed
    - Delayed-release doxylamine succinate 10 mg – pyridoxine hydrochloride 10 mg (Diclectin) may be given for patients with problems with more prolonged nausea during pregnancy [59]
  - Analgesic
    - Acetaminophen 650 mg PO/PR every 6 h as needed
    - Hydrocodone 10 mg (Vicodin, Norco) PO 1/2–1 tablet every 6 h as needed (prescribe no more than 15 tablets)
  - Rescue therapy
    - Prednisone 20 mg tablet PO twice daily for 5 days
    - Intranasal 4% lidocaine (needs to be compounded) 10–20 drops (0.5–1 mL) into nostril on side of the headache while lying on the back with neck extended; may be repeated in 2 min, if needed

IM = intramuscular; IV = intravenous; PO = oral; PR = rectal; SQ = subcutaneous

Anti-emetics During Pregnancy

Anti-emetics most commonly prescribed by practicing obstetricians are promethazine (Phenergan) and ondansetron (Zofran) [31] (see Table 6.4). Ondansetron is preferred for nausea treatment, due to the superior tolerability (e.g., less frequent occurrence of akathisia and sedation) and its designation as an FDA risk-category B drug. Availability as a generic product has reduced cost considerations with ondansetron.

Metoclopramide (Reglan) and prochlorperazine (Compazine) may also be used. As with nonpregnant patients, some women treated with intravenous metoclopramide or prochlorperazine develop akathisia. If present, this requires additional treatment with intravenous diphenhydramine (Benadryl). Although trimethobenzamide (Tigan) is an FDA pregnancy risk-category C drug, limited human data have suggested possible increased risk of congenital anomalies with trimethobenzamide exposure, supporting cautious and limited use during pregnancy.

> ***Pearl for the practitioner:***
> Ondansetron is the preferred ED anti-emetic when pregnant. Ondansetron may be administered intravenously or intramuscularly.

Table 6.4 Preferred medications for ED headache during pregnancy

Drug	Dose	Comments
Safer anti-emetics (FDA risk-category B)		
Ondansetron (Emeset, Emetron, Ondemet, Zofran)	4–8 mg IV over 2–5 min. May use IM if poor venous access	Well tolerated Preferred by obstetricians Also available as orally dissolvable tablet
Metoclopramide (Reglan)	10–20 mg IV	More effective than hydromorphone alone [62]. Metoclopramide 20 mg IV shown to be as effective as SQ sumatriptan (Imitrex) [63]. Watch for akathisia and treat with FDA risk category B drug diphenhydramine (Benadryl) 25 mg IV
Anti-emetics to consider when benefits > potential risks (FDA risk-category C)		
Promethazine (Phenergan, Promethegan)	12.5–25 mg IM	Both anti-emetic and anithistamine components may improve migraine. Watch for akathisia
Droperidol (Inapsine)	2.5–5 mg IM	May be more effective in relieving headache pain than prochlorperazine [64]. As effective as opioid [65]. Black box warning for QT prolongation; not recommended
Prochlorperazine (Compazine)	10 mg IV slowly	As effective for migraine as metoclopramide (Reglan) [66]. Watch for akathisia. Co-administer with diphenhydramine
Trimethobenzamide (Tigan)	200 mg IM	Limited human data suggests possible increased risk of congenital anomalies. Use cautiously. Co-administer with diphenhydramine
Safer pain medications (FDA risk-category B)		
Magnesium sulfate	1–2 g IV	As effective as metoclopramide [35]
Pain medication to consider when benefits > potential risks (FDA risk-category C)		
Tramadol (Ultram)	100 mg IM	Similar efficacy to IM NSAID in non-pregnant patients [67]. Not readily available at all centers
Hydromorphone (Dilaudid)	1–2 mg IM or SQ 0.5–1 mg IV over 2–3 min	Avoid prolonged use. Use at term may result in neonatal respiratory depression

FDA risk-category B=probably safe; studies in animals fail to show adverse fetal effects but human data are lacking; FDA risk-category C=use if benefits warrant possible risk; studies in animals show adverse fetal effects, but human data are lacking

IM intramuscular, *IV* intravenous, *NSAID* nonsteroidal anti-inflammatory drug, *SQ* subcutaneous

Analgesics and Other ED Migraine Treatments During Pregnancy

Analgesics may be used when appropriate during pregnancy (Table 6.4). Useful nonopioid treatment options are often overlooked and ED clinicians move quickly to opioids, which can result in undesirable side effects and inadvertently promoting repeat ED visits or drug-seeking behavior.

Nonsteroidal anti-inflammatory drugs are typically limited to the second trimester of pregnancy, as early first trimester exposure has been linked to increased risk of early miscarriage [32] and third trimester use to premature closure of the ductus arteriosus [33]. Tramadol is an FDA risk-category C drug that may be considered when necessary, although data on use during pregnancy are limited.

> *Pearl for the practitioner:*
> Limit nonsteroidal anti-inflammatory drugs, like intravenous ketorolac, to the second trimester of pregnancy.

Intravenous magnesium sulfate (1–2 g intravenously) may also be effectively used in the ED treatment of migraine [34]. It is a FDA risk-category B drug, safer during pregnancy. In a randomized, prospective study, 2 g intravenous magnesium sulfate was as effective as 10 mg intravenous metoclopramide and more effective than placebo [35].

> *Pearl for the practitioner:*
> 1–2 mg intravenous magnesium sulfate may safely and effectively treat ED migraine in pregnant women.

Lidocaine is an FDA-B drug considered safe during pregnancy. Lidocaine may be compounded into a 4% nasal solution for intranasal use to treat headache. Randomized, controlled trials using intranasal lidocaine for acute or ED treatment of migraine in nonpregnant patients, however, have produced inconsistent results [36–38]. Pregnant patients were excluded from these trials. Intranasal lidocaine is administered to the patient lying on her back with her head extended over the edge of the bed. A total of 0.5–1 mL of 4% lidocaine (10–20 drops) is slowly dripped into the nostril on the side of the headache, repeating 2 min later if needed.

Rescue Therapy

Opioids may have a greater role in pregnant patients whose access to effective migraine-specific treatments like triptans and dihydroergotamine is restricted. Opioids may be used cautiously as rescue therapy, although a recent study showed that migraine patients treated with opioids in the ED had longer duration visits compared with patients treated with nonopioids, further supporting cautious use in patients with benign headache [39]. Although frequently used to treat migraine in the ED, meperidine (Demerol) should be avoided due to potential risks with accumulation of metabolites, such as normeperidine. For this reason, alternative opioids, such as hydromorphone (Dilaudid), are preferred.

> *Pearl for the practitioner:*
> If parenteral opioids are needed as rescue therapy, avoid meperidine and use hydromorphone instead.

Prednisone is an FDA risk-category B drug, and may be used as rescue therapy when acute ED treatment has failed and disabling migraine is prolonged and unremitting [40]. Providing a short course of prednisone (e.g., 20 mg twice daily for 5 days) can help resolve a prolonged, nonresponsive headache episode. Dexamethasone (Decadron) crosses the placenta and is not preferred in pregnancy.

Trigger point injections or occipital nerve blocks (as described in Chap. 4) can also be performed during pregnancy. During later stages of pregnancy, women may be more comfortable leaning over with their head on the exam table during the procedure rather than the prone position.

While many herbal therapies are restricted during pregnancy, topical peppermint oil has been shown to reduce pain, including headache, and may be used during pregnancy. Peppermint oil is derived from the plant *Mentha piperita*, with the main active components being menthol and menthon. A double-blind, placebo-controlled study comparing acute migraine treatment with a 10% ethanol solution of menthol and placebo showed that migraine improved by at least half in 58% with topical menthol compared with only 17% using an inactive placebo ($P=0.0001$) [41]. Migraine pain was completely eliminated for 38% with topical menthol compared vs. 12% with placebo ($P=0.001$).

Treating Migraine During Lactation

Preferred medications for migraine in women who are nursing are described in Table 6.5. A checklist describing typical migraine treatment options for breastfeeding women is provided in Box 6.4.

Table 6.5 Preferred ED headache treatment during lactation

First choice	Second choice	Other
Nonmedication therapies	Magnesium sulfate	Occipital nerve blocks
Rehydration		Trigger point injections
Ketorolac (Toradol)		Valproate (Depacon) if reliable contraception
Sumatriptan (Imitrex)		Hydromorphone (Dilaudid) as rescue therapy
Ondansetron (Zofran)		

Box 6.4 ED Headache Treatment Options During Lactation (Adapted from Marcus DA, Bain PA. Effective migraine treatment in pregnant and lactating women. New York: Springer; 2009)

- Urgent care/ED treatments

  - Ice pack, massage, neck stretches
  - Reduced lights, reduced noise, soothing music
  - Intravenous rehydration
  - Anti-emetic
    - IV ondansetron (Zofran) 4–8 mg over 2–5 min
  - Analgesic
    - Ketorolac (Toradol) 30 mg IV or 60 mg IM
    - SQ sumatriptan (Imitrex) 3–6 mg (efficacy is similar with 3 and 6 mg, with patients preferring the lower dosage)
    - IV sodium valproate (Depacon) 500 mg diluted in 10 mL saline and administered over 5–15 min if reliable contraception is ensured
    - Hydromorphone (Dilaudid) 1–2 mg IM/SQ or 0.5–1.0 mg IV over 2–3 min every 2 h, as needed
    - Occipital nerve blocks
    - Trigger point injections
    - IV dexamethasone (Decadron) 4 mg

- Discharge medication recommendations

  - Anti-emetic
    - Ondansetron (Zofran) 4–8 mg tablets, 1/2–1 tablet every 6 h as needed for severe nausea (patients may prefer orally dissolvable tablets)
  - Analgesic
    - Ibuprofen (Motrin) 600 mg PO every 6 h as needed
    - Naproxen (Anaprox, Naprosyn, Aleve) 500/550 mg PO every 12 h as needed
    - Sumatriptan (Imitrex) 6 mg SQ; or sumatriptan 100 mg PO 1/2–1 tablet, repeated once in 2 h if needed
  - Rescue
    - Prednisone 20 mg twice daily for 5 days

IM = intramuscular; IV = intravenous; PO = oral; SQ = subcutaneous

Anti-emetics During Lactation

Data on drug excretion into breast milk and safe use with nursing are limited for most anti-emetics. The American Gastroenterological Association recently published literature-based recommendations for the use of anti-emetics during lactation, with ondansetron the preferred anti-emetic when nursing [42]. Among those anti-emetics typically used as adjunctive migraine treatment, limited human data with nursing were available for metoclopramide (Reglan), with no human data for ondansetron (Zofran), prochlorperazine (Compazine), and promethazine (Phenergan). Both metoclopramide and prochlorperazine were considered to have potential toxicity, though metoclopramide has a low milk-to-plasma ratio and is considered the safer of the two. The American Academy of Pediatrics advises that metoclopramide should be used with caution [68]. While ondansetron and promethazine are considered to be probably compatible with breastfeeding, there is concern with promethazine. A black box warning against using promethazine in pediatric patients <2 years old suggests caution with nursing may also be warranted. For this reason, the preferred anti-emetic during lactation is ondansetron.

> *Pearl for the practitioner:*
> Intravenous or intramuscular ondansetron is the preferred ED anti-emetic when breastfeeding.

Analgesics and Other ED Migraine Treatments During Lactation

Nonsteroidal anti-inflammatory medications generally have a low milk-to-plasma ratio [43, 44, 68]. Therefore, intravenous ketorolac can be safely used while nursing [68]. Data on effects of tramadol in the nursing baby are limited, with women often recommended to pump and discard milk after exposure, supplementing the next feeding with stored milk. A study evaluating the effects of tramadol administered to 75 breastfeeding women days 2–4 after delivery showed a low drug dose in the infants, with no significant behavioral effects [45].

> *Pearl for the practitioner:*
> Ketorolac is compatible with nursing and is a good first-line treatment due to its low milk-to-plasma ratio.

Nursing patients can also be treated with subcutaneous sumatriptan [68]. Single dose sumatriptan results in minimal drug excretion into the breast milk, so there is no reason to disrupt breastfeeding after dosing with sumatriptan [46].

Intravenous sodium valproate can be used in nursing mothers using reliable contraception [47]. Intravenous magnesium sulfate (1–2 g intravenously) may also be used during lactation.

> **Pearl for the practitioner:**
> Though not recommended during pregnancy, subcutaneous sumatriptan may be safely used when lactating.

Anesthetic therapies, trigger point injections, and occipital nerve blocks, may also be used during breastfeeding.

Topical peppermint oil is theoretically safe to use when nursing, however, it should never be applied to or near the faces of infants or small children, as this may result in serious and potentially life-threatening spasm of respiratory structures and respiratory distress [48].

Treating Cluster Headache During Pregnancy and Lactation

Cluster headache is an uncommon diagnosis in young women. Recommendations for treatment with cluster headache that does occur during pregnancy or when nursing are provided in Box 6.5 [49]. Intranasal lidocaine (FDA risk-category B) administered as a 4% solution with the patient lying down with the head hyperextended is more consistently beneficial for cluster headache than migraine. Anecdotally, intranasal lidocaine has been effective for cluster headache during pregnancy [50].

> **Box 6.5** Cluster Headache Acute Treatment Recommendations When Pregnant or Nursing (Based on [49])
>
> • Oxygen
> • Subcutaneous sumatriptan
> • Intranasal sumatriptan
> • Intranasal lidocaine

Additional Resources for Treating Women During Pregnancy and When Breastfeeding

• *Medications and Mothers' Milk: A Manual of Lactational Pharmacology, 14th edition* by Thomas W. Hale, 2010.

- *Effective Migraine Treatment in Pregnant and Lactating Women: A Practical Guide* by Dawn A. Marcus and Philip A. Bain, 2009.
- *Drugs in Pregnancy and Lactation: A Reference Guide to Fetal and Neonatal Risk, 8th edition* By Gerald G, Briggs, Roger K. Freeman, and Sumner Yaffee, 2008.

Summary

- An appropriate evaluation for potential secondary headaches should not be limited during pregnancy or lactation.
- Safer and effective migraine treatments during pregnancy and lactation include rehydration, anti-emetics (including ondansetron), ketorolac during the second trimester of pregnancy and when lactating, and intravenous magnesium. Sumatriptan may also be used in lactating women. Intravenous sodium valproate may be considered in nonpregnant, nursing women using reliable contraception.
- Opioids should be reserved as rescue therapy when other treatments are ineffective. Additional rescue therapies may include occipital nerve blocks or a short course of prednisone.

References

1. Kelly RH, Russo J, Katon W. Somatic complaints among pregnant women cared for in obstetrics: normal pregnancy or depressive and anxiety symptom amplification revisited? Gen Hosp Psychiatry. 2011;23:107–13.
2. Melhado EM, Maciel JA, Guerreiro CM. Headache during gestation: evaluation of 1101 women. Can J Neurol Sci. 2007;34:187–92.
3. Goldszmidt E, Chettle C, Kern R, et al. The incidence and etiology of postpartum headaches. Can J Anesth. 2004;51:A59.
4. Douglas KA, Redman CW. Eclampsia in the United Kingdom. BMJ. 1994;309:1395–400.
5. Callaghan N. The migraine syndrome in pregnancy. Neurology. 1968;18:197–9.
6. Granella F, Sances G, Zanferrari C, et al. Migraine without aura and reproductive life events: a clinical epidemiological study in 1300 women. Headache. 1993;33:385–9.
7. Chen TC, Leviton A. Headache recurrences in pregnant women with migraine. Headache. 1994;34:107–10.
8. Maggiono F, Alessi C, Maggino T, et al. Primary headaches and pregnancy. Cephalalgia. 1995;15:54.
9. Marcus DA, Scharff L, Turk DC. Longitudinal prospective study of headache during pregnancy and postpartum. Headache. 1999;39:625–32.
10. Sances G, Granella F, Nappi RE, et al. Course of migraine during pregnancy and postpartum: a prospective study. Cephalalgia. 2003;23:197–205.
11. Manzoni GC, Micieli G, Granella F, et al. Cluster headache in women: clinical findings and relationship with reproductive life. Cephalalgia. 1988;8:37–44.
12. van Vliet JA, Favier I, Helmerhorst FM, Haan J, Ferrari MD. Cluster headache in women: relation with menstruation, use of oral contraceptives, pregnancy, and menopause. J Neurol Neurosurg Psychiatry. 2006;77:690–2.

13. Davis LE. Normal laboratory values of CSF during pregnancy. Arch Neurol. 1979;36:443.
14. Kanal E, Barkovich AJ, Bell C, et al. ACR guidance document for safe MR practices: 2007. AJR Am J Roentgenol. 2007;188:1447–74.
15. Levine D, Barnes PD, Edleman RR. Obstetric MR imaging. Radiology. 1999;211:609–17.
16. Baker P, Johnson I, Harvey P, Mansfield P. A three-year follow-up of children imaged in utero using echo-planar magnetic resonance. Am J Obstet Gynecol. 1994;170:32–3.
17. Kanal E, Gillen J, Evans J, Savitz D, Shellock F. Survey of reproductive health among female MR workers. Radiology. 1993;187:395–9.
18. Patel SJ, Reede DL, Katz DS, Subramaniam R, Amorosa JK. Imaging the pregnant patient for nonobstetric conditions: algorithms and radiation dose considerations. Radiography. 2007;27:1705–22.
19. American College of Obstetricians and Gynaecologists Committee Opinion. Guidelines for diagnostic imaging during pregnancy. Obstet Gynecol. 2004;104:647–51.
20. Lowe SA. Diagnostic radiography in pregnancy: risks and reality. Aust N Z J Obstet Gynaecol. 2004;44:191–6.
21. McCollough CH, Schueler BA, Atwell TD, et al. Radiation exposure and pregnancy: when should we be concerned? Radiographics. 2007;27:909–18.
22. Dineen R, Banks A, Lenthall R. Imaging of acute neurological conditions in pregnancy and the puerperium. Clin Radiol. 2005;60:1156–70.
23. Webb JW, Thomsen HS, Morcos SK. The use of iodinated and gadolinium contrast media during pregnancy and lactation. Eur Radiol. 2005;15:1234–40.
24. Patel SJ, Reede DL, Katz DS, Subramaniam R, Amorosa JK. Imaging the pregnant patient for nonobstetric conditions: algorithms and radiation dose considerations. Radiographics. 2007;27:1705–22.
25. Ramachandren S, Cross BJ, Liebeskind DS. Emergent headaches during pregnancy: correlation between neurologic examination and neuroimaging. Am J Neuroradiol. 2007;28:1085–7.
26. Addis A, Sharabi S, Bonati M. Risk classification systems for drug use during pregnancy. Are they a reliable source of information? Drug Saf. 2000;23:245–53.
27. Schreyer P, Sherman DJ, Ervin MG, Day L, Ross MG. Maternal dehydration: impact on ovine amniotic fluid volume and composition. J Dev Physiol. 1990;13:283–7.
28. Urbanski PK. How does hydration affect preterm labor? AWHONN Lifelines. 1997;1:25.
29. Skidmore FM, Williams LS, Fradkin KD, Alonso RJ, Biller J. Presentation, etiology, and outcome of stroke in pregnancy and puerperium. J Stroke Cerebrovasc Dis. 2001;10:1–10.
30. Agnew CL, Ross MG, Fujino Y, et al. Maternal/fetal dehydration: prolonged effects and responses to oral hydration. Am J Physiol. 1993;264:R197–203.
31. Power ML, Milligan LA, Schulkin J. Managing nausea and vomiting of pregnancy: a survey of obstetrician-gynecologists. J Reprod Med. 2007;52:922–8.
32. Evers S, Áfra J, Frese A, et al. EFNS guideline on the drug treatment of migraine – report of an EFNS task force. Eur J Neurol. 2006;13:560–72.
33. Koren G, Florescu A, Costei AM, Boskovic R, Moretti ME. Nonsteroidal antiinflammatory drugs during third trimester and the risk of premature closure of the ductus arteriosus: a meta-analysis. Ann Pharmacother. 2006;40:824–9.
34. Bigal ME, Bordini CA, Tepper SJ, Speciali JG. Intravenous magnesium sulphate in the acute treatment of migraine without aura and migraine with aura. A randomized, double-blind, placebo-controlled study. Cephalalgia. 2002;22:345–53.
35. Cete Y, Dora B, Ertan C, Ozdemir C, Oktay C. A randomized prospective placebo-controlled study of intravenous magnesium sulphate vs. metoclopramide in the management of acute migraine attacks in the Emergency Department. Cephalalgia. 2005;25:199–204.
36. Maizels M, Scott B, Cohen W, Chen W. Intranasal lidocaine for treatment of migraine: a randomized, double-blind, controlled trial. JAMA. 1996;276:319–21.
37. Maizels M, Geiger AM. Intranasal lidocaine for migraine: a randomized trial and open-label follow-up. Headache. 1999;39:543–51.

38. Blanda M, Rench T, Gerson LW, Weigand JV. Intranasal lidocaine for the treatment of migraine headache: a randomized, controlled trial. Acad Emerg Med. 2001;8:337–42.
39. Tornabene SV, Deutsch R, Davis DP, Chan TC, Vilke GM. Evaluating the use and timing of opioids for the treatment of migraine headaches in the emergency department. J Emerg Med. 2009;36:333–7.
40. Von Seggern RL, Adelman JU. Practice and economics cost considerations in headache treatment. Part 2: acute migraine treatment. Headache. 1996;36:493–502.
41. Borhani Haghighi A, Motazedian S, Rezaii R, et al. Cutaneous application of menthol 10% solution as an abortive treatment of migraine without aura: a randomised, double-blind, placebo-controlled, crossed-over study. Int J Clin Pract. 2010;64:451–6.
42. Mahadevan U, Kane S. American gastroenterological association institute medical position statement on the use of gastrointestinal medications in pregnancy. Gastroenterology. 2006; 131:283–311.
43. Beaulac-Baillargeon L, Allard G. Distribution of indomethacin in human milk and estimation of its mil to plasma ratio in vitro. Br J Clin Pharmacol. 1993;36:413–6.
44. Gardiner SJ, Doogue MP, Zhang M, Begg EJ. Quantification of infant exposure to celecoxib through breast milk. Br J Clin Pharmacol. 2006;61:101–4.
45. Ilett KF, Paech MJ, Page-Sharp M, et al. Use of a sparse sampling study design to assess transfer of tramadol and its O-desmethyl metabolite into transitional breast milk. Br J Clin Pharmacol. 2008;65:661–6.
46. Wojnar-Horton RE, Hackett LP, et al. Distribution and excretion of sumatriptan in human milk. Br J Clin Pharmacol. 1996;41:217–21.
47. Waberzinek G, Marková J, Mastík J. Safety and efficacy of intravenous sodium valproate in the treatment of acute migraine. Neuro Endocrinol Lett. 2007;28:59–64.
48. Kligler B, Chaudhary S. Peppermint oil. Am Fam Phys. 2007;75:1027–30.
49. Jürgens TP, Schaefer C, May A. Treatment of cluster headache in pregnancy and lactation. Cephalalgia. 2009;29:391–400.
50. Giraud P, Chauvet S. Cluster headache during pregnancy: case report and literature review. Headache. 2009;49:136–9.
51. Simbar M, Karimian Z, Afrakhteh M, Akbarzadeh A, Kouchaki E. Increased risk of pre-eclampsia (PE) among women with the history of migraine. Clin Exp Hypertens. 2010;32: 159–65.
52. Panagariya A, Maru A. Cerebral venous thrombosis in pregnancy and puerperium – a prospective study. J Assoc Physicians India. 1997;45:857–9.
53. Azpilcueta A, Peral C, Giraldo I, Chen FJ, Contreras G. Meningioma in pregnancy. Report of a case and review of the literature. Ginecol Obstet Mex. 1995;63:349–51.
54. Saitoh Y, Oku Y, Izumoto S, Go J. Rapid growth of a meningioma during pregnancy: relationship with estrogen and progesterone receptors – case report. Neurol Med Chir (Tokyo). 1989;29:440–3.
55. Arseni C, Simoca I, Jipescu I, Leventi E, Grecu P, Sima A. Pseudotumor cerebri: risk factors, clinical course, prognostic criteria. Rom J Neurol Psychiatry. 1992;30:115–32.
56. Katz VL, Peterson R, Cefalo RC. Pseudotumor cerebri and pregnancy. Am J Perinatol. 1989;6:442–5.
57. Koontz WL, Herbert WP, Cefalo RC. Pseudotumor cerebri in pregnancy. Obstet Gynecol. 1983;62:324–7.
58. Evans RW, Lee AG. Idiopathic intracranial hypertension in pregnancy. Headache. 2010;50: 1513–5.
59. Koren G, Clark S, Hankins GD, et al. Effectiveness of delayed-release doxylamine and pyridoxine for nausea and vomiting of pregnancy: a randomized placebo controlled trial. Am J Obstet Gynecol. 2010;203:571.e1–7.
60. Coutinho JM, Ferro JM, Canhão P, et al. Cerebral venous and sinus thrombosis in women. Stroke. 2009;40:2356–61.
61. Rodriguez-Thompson D, Lieberman ES. Use of a random urinary protein-to-creatinine ratio for the diagnosis of significant proteinuria during pregnancy. Am J Obstet Gynecol. 2001;185:808–11.

62. Griffith JD, Mycyk MB, Kyriacou DN. Metoclopramide versus hydromorphone for the emergency department treatment of migraine headache. J Pain. 2008;9:88–94.
63. Friedman BW, Corbo J, Lipton RB, et al. A trial of metoclopramide vs sumatriptan for the emergency department treatment of migraines. Neurology. 2005;64:463–8.
64. Miner JR, Fish SJ, Smith SW, Biros MH. Droperidol vs. prochlorperazine for benign headaches in the emergency department. Acad Emerg Med. 2001;8:873–9.
65. Richman PB, Allegra J, Eskin B, et al. A randomized clinical trial to assess the efficacy of intramuscular droperidol for the treatment of acute migraine headache. Am J Emerg Med. 2002;20:39–42.
66. Friedman BW, Esses D, Solorzano C, et al. Evaluating the use and timing of opioids for the treatment of migraine headaches in the emergency department. Ann Emerg Med. 2008;52:399–406.
67. Engindeniz Z, Demircan C, Karli N, et al. Intramuscular tramadol vs. diclofenac sodium for the treatment of acute migraine attacks in emergency department: a prospective, randomised, double-blind study. J Headache Pain. 2005;6:143–8.
68. American Academy of Pediatric Committee on Drugs. The transfer of drugs and other chemicals into human milk. Pediatrics. 2001;108:776–89.

Chapter 7
Treatment of the Older Adult Patient (>50 Years Old) with Acute Headache in the ED

Key Chapter Points:

- Primary headaches are more common in younger than older adult patients.
- Adults >50 years old presenting to the ED with headache will require a more detailed evaluation for secondary headache than younger adults.
- Common secondary headaches in adults >50 years old may include a wide range of disorders, including vascular conditions, acute angle-closure glaucoma, medication side effects, carbon monoxide poisoning, primary and metastatic neoplasm, infection, and trauma.
- Giant cell arteritis is a medical emergency requiring definitive, presumptive treatment initiation in the ED.

Keywords Cognitive loss • Giant cell arteritis • Hypnic headache • Subdural hematoma

---

Case 1

Anna is a 73-year-old with a life-long history of migraines. She is otherwise healthy except for atrial fibrillation treated with warfarin and hypercholesterolemia treated with a statin. She reports having debilitating migraine attacks every couple of weeks, especially when she travels or there is a change in the weather. High stress also aggravates her headaches. Usually she treats her headaches with over-the-counter analgesics and sinus medications, with fair relief. Her headaches usually resolve within about 12 h. Anna came to the ED for a problematic headache that started 1½ days ago. She came to the ED because she has her children and grandchildren visiting and was "looking for a stronger pain medication to knock out my headache so the headache wouldn't spoil the kids' visit." Anna reported no other complaints or trauma. Anna's

---

(continued)

(continued)

D.A. Marcus and P.A. Bain, *Practical Assessment and Treatment of the Patient with Headaches in the Emergency Department and Urgent Care Clinic*, DOI 10.1007/978-1-4614-0002-8_7, © Springer Science+Business Media, LLC 2011

Case 1 (continued)

daughter arrived at the end of the history and commented to the doctor that she was surprised how her mother seemed to have gotten more forgetful since her last visit. She also reminded her mother to mention the lump on her head that she got the previous day after missing a step going down the stairs and bumping her head against the wall.

Not unexpectedly, an imaging study revealed that Anna had suffered a subdural hematoma after her seemingly minor trauma, likely aggravated by her anticoagulation therapy. This case highlights the importance of recognizing a change in a stable headache pattern as an indication for additional investigation, particularly in the older patient. Furthermore, this case also shows the need to complete mental status screening in all older patients to ensure the accuracy of historical information and to enlist impressions of family members, caregivers, and others in close contact with the patient to help identify important changes that might suggest a secondary headache.

New headache or a change in a chronic headache pattern occurring in an adult >50 years old needs a more detailed work-up to rule out secondary causes of headache than might be necessary for younger adults [1]. For example, a report of cerebrovascular disease in elderly patients found that one in three patients with an acute intracerebral hemorrhage had early symptoms of headache [2]. Furthermore, headache is one of the most common side effects reported with medications, so a new drug or change in medication regimen also needs to be considered. For example, among men using sildenafil citrate (Viagra), 11–18% report a side effect of headache [3, 4]. Often the presence of additional symptoms or signs, such as a history of minor trauma for patients with a subdural hematoma, similar headache in other family members for patients with carbon monoxide poisoning, neurological deficits in patients with intracranial pathology, or marked conjunctival injection in patients with acute angle-closure glaucoma, provide important diagnostic clues for older patients with secondary headaches (Table 7.1) [5].

Table 7.1 Headache emergencies in seniors

Category	Disorders
Vascular	Subarachnoid hemorrhage
	Subdural hematoma
	Giant cell arteritis
	Cerebrovascular accident
Ophthalmologic	Acute angle-closure glaucoma
Toxic	Medication side effects
	Carbon monoxide poisoning
Neoplastic	Primary brain tumor
	Metastatic disease
Infectious	Encephalitis
	Meningitis
	Brain abscess

Pearl for the practitioner:
Secondary headaches caused by serious pathology occur in 2% of all people attending the ED for nontraumatic headache, but 6% of adults ≥50 years old and 11% of seniors ≥75 years old [1].

Assessment for Comorbid Cognitive Dysfunction

A recent survey of emergency department (ED) patients ≥65 years old identified cognitive dysfunction in 35% of patients, although only 6% had a pre-existing diagnosis noted in their record [6]. In this study, over one-third of all seniors coming to the ED were excluded because they had received sedating medication and were, therefore, ineligible for participating. Ensuring reliable reporting by assessing mental status is an essential part of the ED evaluation of the senior with headache. Tools to quickly screen for cognitive dysfunction that have been validated in the ED are provided in Boxes 7.1 and 7.2 [6–8]. Patients with identified cognitive dysfunction that had not been previously recognized by family or caregivers need additional evaluation to rule out acute pathology.

Pearl for the practitioner:
Cognitive dysfunction in older adults is more common than expected, affecting up to one in three seniors seen in the ED. Asking several pointed questions can help identify patients with likely cognitive dysfunction in the ED.

Box 7.1 Six-Item Screener

This tool is a sensitive, brief cognitive assessment tool that has been validated in the ED. Questions are asked of a reliable caregiver. False-positive rate, however, is 23% (reprinted with permission from [6]).

Instructions to the patient: I would like to ask you some questions that may ask you to use your memory. I am going to name three objects. Please wait until I say all three words, then repeat them. Remember these words for me: GRASS – PAPER – SHOE. (May repeat names 3 times if necessary, repetition not scored).

1. What year is this?
2. What month is this?
3. What is the day of the week?
4. After one-minute. What are the three objects that I asked you to remember?
5. [Grass]

(continued)

Box 7.1 (continued)
6. [Paper]
7. [Shoe]

Each correct response is awarded one-point. Two of more errors is considered high-risk for cognitive impairment.

Box 7.2 AD8 Dementia Screener Patient Interview

The AD8 has been validated in the ED. This tool can be used when a caregiver is not available to answer questions about the patient. These questions are asked directly to the patient (adapted from [7]).

Have you noticed a change in any of the following over that last several years:

1. Problems making decisions, problems with thinking, or making bad financial decisions?
2. Loss of interest in hobbies or other activities?
3. Repeating the same questions, stories, or statements over and over?
4. Trouble learning to use tools, appliances, or electronic gadgets, like computers, remote controls, or microwaves?
5. Forgetting the correct month of the year?
6. Trouble balancing the checkbook, paying income taxes, or paying bills?
7. Trouble remembering appointments?
8. Daily problems with your thinking or memory?

Patients answering "yes" to two or more items are likely to have cognitive impairment.

Traumatic Headache

Age-related cerebral atrophy with subsequent stretching of bridging veins in the dura results in increased risk of subdural in older adults. Acute subdural hemorrhage has been reported in older adults without external trauma, including cases occurring after bouts of coughing [9]. Evidence of trauma may be subtle. Elderly patients may be vulnerable to trauma due to unreported falls, unsteady gait, and elder abuse.

Pearl for the practitioner:
Traumatic headache should always be considered in the evaluation of an older adult presenting to the ED with headache.

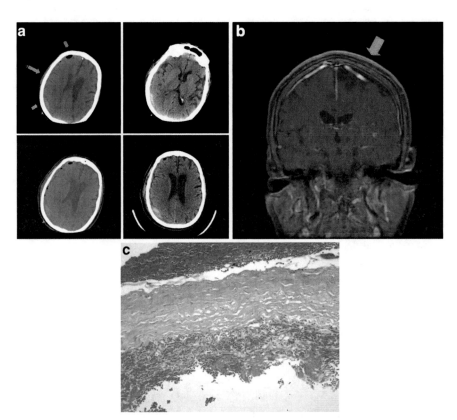

Fig. 7.1 Subdural hemorrhage (images courtesy of Clayton A. Wiley, MD, PhD). (**a**) Images with CT, horizontal view. These scans were taken from an elderly patient after a fall. At 7 o'clock there is an ellipse of bright signal between the skull and brain (*pink arrow*). At 11 o'clock there is a dark air bubble, which is the result of drainage of a hematoma from the front of the brain (*green arrow*). The *dashed, yellow arrow* points to exterior bruising and an external hematoma caused by the patient's fall. (**b**) Magnetic resonance imaging, coronal view. This coronal plane image demonstrates a dark collection of blood on the right side of the image on the surface of the brain (*yellow arrow*). The ventricle on that side is mildly compressed, consistent with the mass effect of the overlying blood clot. (**c**) Pathology findings. This lower power image is of a hematoxylin (*blue*) and eosin (*red*) stained section from the dense connective tissue (*pink*) covering the brain. A collection of dark red blood is seen on the surface of the dura

Typical neuroimaging and pathologic findings of subdural hemorrhage are shown in Fig. 7.1. Patients with subdural hematomas often present with headache, confusion, ataxia, and/or hemiparesis. Because of this, subdural hematomas can mimic a variety of other neurological conditions that affect older adults, including dementia, stroke, neoplasm, and normal pressure hydrocephalus.

Mortality from acute subdural hematoma in the elderly is high, with a poor prognosis predicted by: [10]

• Glasgow Coma Scale score 3–8;
• Pupillary abnormalities;
• Contusions and subarachnoid hemorrhage seen on imaging;

- Midline brain shift on imaging larger than the thickness of the subdural hematoma;
- Elevated intracranial pressure >40 mmHg.

Patients with acute subdural hematomas with focal neurologic signs should be urgently evaluated by neurosurgery. In some cases, when the subdural is small and neurological deficits are absent, conservative treatment with close follow-up and serial imaging may be appropriate [11].

Nontraumatic Headache

A wide range of secondary, nontraumatic headaches (see Chap. 3) occur more commonly in older adults, including headache caused by

- Acute angle-closure glaucoma;
- Acute stroke;
- Carbon monoxide poisoning;
- Malignancy (primary and metastatic);
- Medication side effects.

As in younger patients, infections are another common cause of secondary, nontraumatic headache in older adults. As patient age increases, the likelihood of headache being caused by a secondary headache becomes more likely. Patients >50 years old diagnosed with a presumptive primary headache should always have close follow-up with their primary care provider arranged for further evaluation to ensure a secondary headache was not missed.

Giant Cell Arteritis

Giant cell arteritis (temporal arteritis) is an inflammatory condition experienced as head pain or scalp tenderness, often associated with fatigue with chewing, visual disturbance, and low-grade fever. Giant cell arteritis may occur as an isolated head pain syndrome or be associated with polymyalgia rheumatica (Case 2 and Table 7.2) [12].

Giant cell arteritis is considered to be a medical emergency due to significant risk for permanent visual loss in untreated patients. Visual symptoms occur in 30% of patients with biopsy-proven giant cell arteritis, with permanent partial or total visual loss occurring in 19%, most commonly due to anterior ischemic neuropathy (92%) and less commonly central retinal artery occlusion (8%) [13]. Visual loss is unilateral for three of every four patients. Stroke, usually in the vertebrobasilar distribution, occurs in approximately 3% of giant cell arteritis patients [14].

Giant cell arteritis should be considered in the differential diagnosis of any new headache in patients >50 years old because of the significant risk for vision loss and stroke (Fig. 7.2). Initial evaluation and presumptive treatment should be started in the ED. Typical positive biopsy findings with giant cell arteritis are shown in Fig. 7.3.

Table 7.2 Prevalence of symptoms in patients with giant cell arteritis or polymyalgia rheumatica (based on [12])

Giant cell arteritis		Polymyalgia rheumatica	
Symptom	% Patients	Symptom	% Patients
Head pain/scalp tenderness	66	Giant cell arteritis	16–21
Fatigue with chewing (jaw claudication)	50	Shoulder pain and stiffness	70–95
Polymyalgia rheumatica	40	Hip and neck pain and stiffness	50–70
Visual loss/disturbance	20	Distal extremity symptoms (e.g., asymmetrical arthritis in the wrists and knees, carpal tunnel syndrome, hand and foot edema)	50
Low grade fever	15	Systemic symptoms (e.g., anorexia, fatigue, fever, weight loss)	30
Cough	10		

Case 2

Joe is a 76-year-old man who presents to the ED with a 3-week history of bilateral headache over the sides of his head and temples. "I think I've had the flu. I've had a bit of a low-grade fever and aching in both of my shoulders. Even my jaw hurts when I chew. Nothing is helping this headache and I came to the ED because I just can't take it anymore!"

Joe's general medical and neurological examinations are unremarkable except for tenderness over his right temple. Because of his age and symptoms, a non-contrasted brain CT and blood work, including a erythrocyte sedimentation rate (ESR) are performed. Everything is unremarkable except for his ESR, which is 93 mm/h. Joe was presumptively diagnosed with giant cell arteritis, treated with steroids, and scheduled for a temporal artery biopsy and follow-up the next day with this primary care provider.

Pearl for the practitioner:

Giant cell arteritis is a medical emergency that should be considered in all patients >50 years old with an unexplained, new onset headache that cannot be attributed to other conditions. Diagnosis is strengthened by elevated inflammatory markers and a dramatic symptomatic improvement with steroids. Biopsy may be negative in giant cell arteritis because inflammatory changes typically don't affect all parts of the blood vessel and may be missed in sampling. Referral to a rheumatologist is helpful when the diagnosis is in doubt.

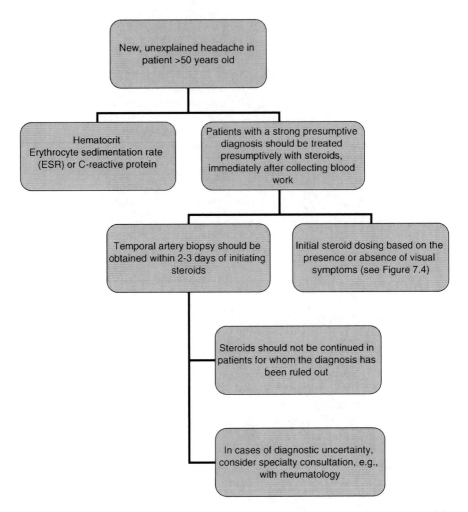

Fig. 7.2 Emergency assessment and treatment of possible giant cell arteritis. As discussed in Chap. 2, C-reactive protein is a more sensitive marker for giant cell arteritis than erythrocyte sedimentation rate

Glucocorticoids are first-line treatment for giant cell arteritis, effectively relieving clinical symptoms and preventing ischemic complications in most patients (Fig. 7.4) [15]. The ED provider should begin empiric steroids and arrange for close follow-up by the patient's primary care doctor, neurologist, or rheumatologist. Temporal artery biopsy is generally scheduled soon after the presumptive diagnosis has been made, generally within days to 2 weeks. Biopsy of one or both of the temporal arteries should be done within 1–2 weeks to maximize the yield of the biopsy, although treatment should not be delayed while waiting for a biopsy. Subsequent steroid tapering depends on continuation of symptomatic control and reduction in inflammatory markers. Small increases in inflammatory markers often occur during steroid

Fig. 7.3 Giant cell arteritis (images courtesy of Clayton A. Wiley, MD, PhD). Hematoxylin (*blue*) and eosin (*red*) stained section from the temporal artery of a patient with giant cell arteritis. (**a**) Low-power view. This lower power image shows the artery lumen severely narrowed, compromising the ability to conduct blood to the tissues, which may result in visual loss and stroke. (**b**) High-power. This high power image shows a collection of blue cells forming a small whorl on the lower left side of the artery wall. This whorl is called a granuloma and represents an inflammatory response to the vessel wall. Such inflammation can compromise the artery lumen and lead to infarction of the tissue dependent upon blood from this vessel

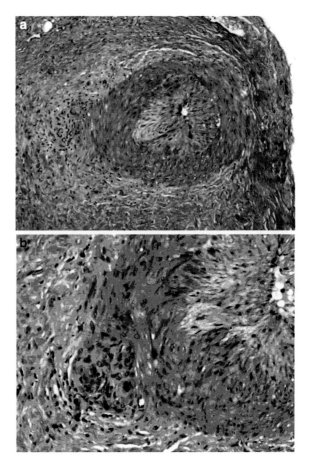

tapering and do not require an increase in steroids if the patient remains asymptomatic. Although treatment is started before a definitive diagnosis is verified, steroid treatment should not be continued in patients for whom the diagnosis has been ruled out as glucocorticoid complications occur frequently (Table 7.3) [16]. Nonsteroid treatments with methotrexate, azathioprine, antitumor necrosis factor-α monoclonal antibody infliximab, and low-dose aspirin have been tested, although controlled trial data are sparse and inconsistent [15].

Rare Hypnic Headache

Hypnic headache is an unusual primary headache that typically occurs in people after 50 years of age. Hypnic headaches occur during sleep and have been dubbed "alarm clock headache" since these short-duration nighttime headaches awaken

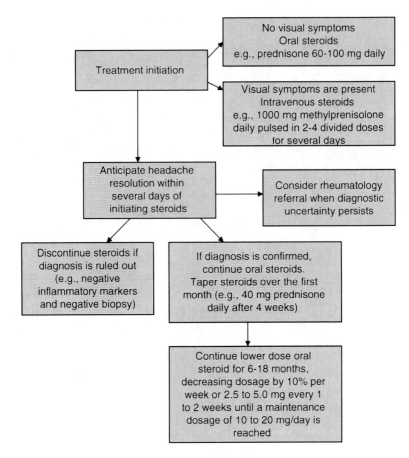

Fig. 7.4 Treatment regimen for giant cell arteritis

Table 7.3 Incidence of steroid-related complications with treatment for giant cell arteritis (based on [16])

Steroid-related complication	Percentage of patients experiencing
Any glucocorticoid side effect	86
Posterior subcapsular cataract	41
Any fracture	38
Vertebral fracture	23
Hip fracture	16
Infection	31
Hypertension	22
Diabetes	9
Gastrointestinal bleeding	4

Box 7.3 Hypnic Headache Characteristics

- Headache occurs during sleep, often predictably at the same time each night
- Patient experiences ≥15 episodes per month
- Pain is bilateral or diffuse
- Pain lasts a few minutes up to 3 h
- There are no associated autonomic symptoms
- Secondary headache has been excluded

Table 7.4 Typical features of hypnic headache (based on [18])

Characteristic	Number
Mean age at onset	63 years
Female:male ratio	2:1
Pain location (%)	
Unilateral	39
Bilateral	61
Pain description (%)	
Dull	57
Throbbing	38
Sharp or stabbing	5
Pain severity (%)	
Mild	2
Moderate	68
Severe	31

patients predictably from sleep (Box 7.3). Rapid eye movement (REM) sleep has been identified as a consistent trigger for hypnic headaches [17]. In contrast to strictly unilateral and usually periorbital cluster headaches, the pain of hypnic headache is generally more diffuse and not associated with autonomic features like rhinorrhea or lacrimation. A review of 71 case reports of hypnic headache in the literature resulted in a description of typical features (Table 7.4) [18]. Associated nausea occurred in one in every five patients, with photophobia, phonophobia, and autonomic features reported infrequently.

> *Pearl for the practitioner:*
> Hypnic headache is a rare, primary headache that wakes seniors predictably from dream sleep.

A diagnosis of hypnic headache should only be made after evaluations have ruled out secondary causes of headache. Hypnic-like headache was recently reported in a 58-year-old man diagnosed with cerebellar hemangioblastoma [19]. Hypnic-type headache has previously been reported in patients subsequently diagnosed with other pituitary and posterior fossa pathologies, including stroke and tumor [20–23].

ED treatment of hypnic headache should focus on reassurance and arranging post-ED follow-up. Acute treatment has been successful with acetaminophen [18]. Preventive therapy may be initiated with lithium or indomethacin; however, both require close follow-up due to significant side effects [24]. Patients failing to have hypnic headaches controlled with these therapies may be treated with caffeine and melatonin or flunarizine.

Summary

- About one in every ten older adults presenting to the ED with a nontraumatic headache will be diagnosed with a serious, secondary headache.
- A survey identified cognitive dysfunction in one in three seniors ≥65 years old in the ED.
- Subdural hematomas may occur in elderly patients after only minor trauma.
- Common nontraumatic secondary headaches in older adults include giant cell arteritis, medication side effects, carbon monoxide poisoning, primary and metastatic malignancy, acute angle-closure glaucoma, and infections.
- Giant cell arteritis is a medical emergency requiring presumptive initiation of treatment with steroids in the ED.
- Hypnic headache is a rare, primary headache that occurs like clockwork, typically during dream sleep. Secondary headaches often mimic hypnic headache, so this diagnosis should only be considered after ruling out secondary causes of headache.

References

1. Goldstein JN, Camargo CA, Pelletier AJ, Edlow JA. Headache in the United States emergency departments: demographics, work-up and frequency of pathological disease. Cephalalgia. 2006;26:684–90.
2. Kawahata N. Cerebrovascular disease in the elderly – clinical study of 31 cases with acute intracerebral hemorrhages. Rinsho Shinkeigaku. 1990;30:713–17.
3. Fink HA, MacDonald R, Rutks IR, Nelson DB, Wilt TJ. Sildenafil for male erectile dysfunction: a systematic review and meta-analysis. Arch Intern Med. 2002;162:1349–60.
4. Müller A, Smith L, Parker M, Mulhall JP. Analysis of the efficacy and safety of sildenafil citrate in the geriatric population. BJU Int. 2007;100:117–21.
5. Walker RA, Wadman MC. Headache in the elderly. Clin Geriatr Med. 2007;23:291–305.
6. Carpenter CR, Despain B, Keeling TN, Shah M, Rothenberger M. The Six-Item Screener and AD8 for the detection of cognitive impairment in geriatric emergency department patients. Ann Emerg Med. 2011;57:653–61.
7. Galvin JE, Roe CM, Powlishta KK, et al. The AD8: a brief interview to detect dementia. Neurology. 2005;65:559–64.
8. Galvin JE, Roe CM, Coats MA, Morris JC. Patient's rating of cognitive ability: using the AD8, a brief informant interview, as a self-rating tool to detect dementia. Arch Neurol. 2007;64:725–30.

9. Komatsu Y, Uemura K, Yasuda S, et al. Acute subdural hemorrhage of arterial origin: report of three cases. No Shinkei Geka. 1997;25:841–45.

10. Petridid AK, Dörner L, Doukas A, et al. Acute subdural hematoma in the elderly; clinical and CT factors influencing the surgical treatment decision. Cen Eur Neurosurg. 2009;70:73–8.

11. Karnath B. Subdural hematoma: presentation and management in older adults. Geriatrics. 2004;59:18–23.

12. Salvarani C, Cantini F, Boiardi L, Hunder GG. Medical progress: polymyalgia rheumatica and temporal arteritis. NEJM. 2002;347:261–71.

13. Salvarini C, Cimino L, Macchioni P, et al. Risk factors for visual loss in an Italian population-based cohort of patients with giant cell arteritis. Arthritis Care Res. 2005;53:293–7.

14. Gonzalez-Gay MA, Blanco R, Rodriguez-Valverde V, et al. Permanent visual loss and cerebro-vascular accidents in giant cell arteritis. Arthritis Rheum. 1998;41:1497–504.

15. Pipitone N, Salvarani C. Improving therapeutic options for patients with giant cell arteritis. Curr Opin Rheumatol. 2008;20:17–22.

16. Proven A, Gabriel SE, Orces C, O'Fallon M, Hunder GG. Glucocorticoid therapy in giant cell arteritis: duration and adverse outcomes. Arthritis Care Res. 2003;49:703–8.

17. De Simone R, Marano E, Ranieri A, Bonavita V. Hypnic headache: an update. Neurol Sci. 2006;27:S144–8.

18. Evers S, Goadsby PJ. Hypnic headache. Clinical features, pathophysiology, and treatment. Neurology. 2003;60:905–9.

19. Mullally WJ, Hall KE. Hypnic headache secondary to haemangioblastoma of the cerebellum. Cephalalgia. 2010;30:887–9.

20. Peatfield RC, Mendoza ND. Posterior fossa meningioma presenting as hypnic headache. Headache. 2003;43:1007–8.

21. Gil-Gouveia R, Goadsby PJ. Secondary 'hypnic headache'. J Neurol. 2007;254:646–54.

22. Valentinis L, Tuniz F, Mucchiut M, et al. Hypnic headache secondary to growth hormone-secreting pituitary tumour. Cephalalgia. 2009;29:82–4.

23. Garza I, Hall K. Symptomatic hypnic headache secondary to nonfunctioning pituitary mac-roadenoma. Headache. 2009;49:470–2.

24. Lisotto C, Rossi P, Tassorelli C, Ferrante E, Nappi G. Focus on therapy of hypnic headache. J Headache Pain. 2010;11:349–54.

Chapter 8
Managing Risk in the ED

Key Chapter Points

- ED physicians ranked 5th in frequency of malpractice claims.
- ED headache is not a diagnosis commonly associated with litigation.
- The "difficult patient" encounter usually occurs because of a combination of patient, healthcare provider, and situational factors.
- Be the BOSS when dealing with patients making unreasonable demands by setting Boundaries, utilizing multiple treatment Options, Scripting responses to common patient concerns, and treating patients with Sincere concern and respect.
- Most errors in diagnosis in the ED stem from errors in thought processes during decision making rather than lack of knowledge.
- Physicians must understand the laws of their state and make sure that their diagnostic approach and approach to informed consent complies with state laws.

Keywords Analgesic overuse headache • Context errors • Drug seeking • Informed consent • Litigation • Malpractice • Metacognition

Working in the emergency department (ED) is challenging – ED patients are complicated, at times suboptimal historians, and occasionally present with symptoms caused by serious, life-threatening conditions. ED personnel have to make critical decisions quickly and expertly, sometimes based on limited information. Furthermore, the time available for diagnosis is limited in the ED and follow-up after ED discharge can be variable. Dealing with ED patients who present with acute headaches can be frustrating for the clinician. Headache patients may have unrealistic expectations for their ED visit. Because of the inherent complexities of the ED (e.g., limited time and access to information for diagnosis, suboptimal historians, lack of follow-up, etc.), risk management is also a concern.

D.A. Marcus and P.A. Bain, *Practical Assessment and Treatment of the Patient* *with Headaches in the Emergency Department and Urgent Care Clinic,* DOI 10.1007/978-1-4614-0002-8_8, © Springer Science+Business Media, LLC 2011

Based on 2007–2008 data from the Physician Insurers Association of America, ED physicians ranked fifth in frequency of malpractice claims after obstetrics/gynecology, general surgery, surgical subspecialties, and radiology (Box 8.1) [1]. A review of claims resulting from an ED visit over a period of 23 years identified 11,529 claims [2]. Four out of five cases were made against non-ED staff who had provided care in the ED, with the largest awards against anesthesiologists, neurologists, and psychiatrists (Box 8.2). Headache did not make the list of top ten diagnoses associated with malpractice claims in the ED.

> *Pearl for the practitioner:*
> About 80% of claims attributed to ED visits are against non-ED staff who provided services to ED patients. Headache is not a common diagnosis associated with ED malpractice claims.

Case 1

Melinda is a 35-year-old female with a long history of headaches. Initially, her headaches were infrequent, disabling attacks associated with nausea and light sensitivity. Over time, her headaches became more frequent and more severe. In the past 5 years, she has had a headache nearly every day with frequent ED visits occurring 3–5 times per month. She presents to the ED today with her usual headache rated "12/10" in severity without any significant nausea. She demands Demerol, telling the doctor, "Demerol is the only thing that has ever worked." Melinda ran out of Vicodin 5 days ago, exceeding the dose instructions from her primary care physician. She insists she "needed more Vicodin because I've been under a lot of stress." The only change in her usual routine was a camping trip in northwest Wisconsin approximately 2–3 weeks earlier that was cut short because of numerous bug bites. On the way home, Melinda was involved in a minor motor vehicle accident. Melinda is very agitated, insisting, "If you'd just give me my Demerol and Vicodin, I could go home and finally get this headache under control! I don't feel well. I have had a low-grade fever for the past week. I just want to go home and go to bed." Melinda and the ED doctor argue about giving her Demerol and Vicodin. Because the ED is overflowing with patients, the ED physician ultimately provides the patient with Demerol IM and 30 Vicodin tablets to go home with. One day after going home from the ED, Melinda suffers a seizure and is brought back to the ED. She has a bull's-eye rash on her back and spinal tap is consistent with Lyme meningitis. Melinda is admitted to the hospital, recovers, and is considering legal action against the ED physician for "missing the diagnosis."

Box 8.1 Malpractice Figures from American Medical Association Analysis of Claims Filed (Based on [1])

- *The bad news*

  - 42% of all physicians report having been sued at some point during their careers
  - 50% of ED doctors have been sued, with 31% sued at least twice
  - The average defense cost per claim was $40,649

- *The good news*

  - 65% of claims were dropped and 30% were settled or resolved through other methods
  - Only 5% of claims were brought to trial
  - Among claims brought to trial, 90% found in favor of the defending doctor
  - A review of closed claims showed no injury occurred in 3% of claims and no error could be identified in an additional 37% of claims

---

Box 8.2 Claims Related to an ED Visit (Based on [2])

- 31% of claims resulted in a payment to the claimant
- 81% of claims were attributed to care received in the ED that was provided by non-ED specialty staff who provided direct care or consultation services to the patient
- 37% of claims were attributed to an error in diagnosis
- Diagnoses most commonly involved in ED litigation were acute myocardial infarction, chest pain, symptoms involving the abdomen and pelvis (including appendicitis), injury to multiple body parts, and fractures

---

Melinda's case illustrates several important points. First, although Melinda has a history of migraine, her current headaches suggest several alternative diagnoses. Patients regularly using acute medications for the management of headache more than 3 days per week are at risk for developing *analgesic overuse headache* (Boxes 8.3 and 8.4), which used to be called *rebound headache* [3, 4]. For these patients, the overuse of prescription or nonprescription analgesics is believed to result in a up-regulation of serotonin receptors in the brain that makes the person more susceptible to headaches [5]. Headaches tend to become more frequent, more severe, and less responsive to treatment. Increasing analgesics escalates the headache problem and patients need to be treated with analgesic medication taper, with headaches usually improving over several weeks to months. Patients with

Box 8.3 Features of Analgesic Overuse Headache

- Patients regularly using acute migraine medication more than 2 days per week for at least 6 weeks are at risk for a worsening of chronic headache
- Analgesic overuse headache typically occurs in patients with underlying headaches, such as migraine or post-traumatic headache
- Regular use of analgesics tends to make headaches more frequent and more severe
- Continuing frequent analgesic use further aggravates analgesic overuse headache
- Medications that can cause analgesic overuse headache include over-the-counter or prescription analgesics (including opioid and non-opioid therapies), ergotamine, and triptans
- Analgesic overuse is less common with nonibuprofen nonsteroidal anti-inflammatory drugs (NSAIDs)
- Treatment requires tapering or discontinuing offending medications. Patients may use limited doses of nonibuprofen NSAIDs or tramadol dosed twice daily during taper and then for occasional severe headaches only after discontinuation of offending medications. Patients may also be treated with standard migraine prevention therapy (e.g., antidepressants [e.g., amitriptyline], beta-blockers [e.g., propranolol], or neuromodulating anti-epileptics [e.g., topiramate])
- Headache frequency and severity typically decrease over weeks to months after analgesic discontinuation. After medication withdrawal, headache frequency decreases by an average of 46% [29]
- Patients and clinicians should be aware that improvement typically takes about 6–8 weeks for most patients, with significant improvement occurring in >80% of patients 4 months after discontinuing overused medications [30]

suspected analgesic overuse headache should be provided with written information to reinforce the doctor's recommendation to limit problematic medications (Box 8.5). Melinda might also have had a new type of headache related to her recent head trauma or other medication conditions, including infection that was suggested by her report of fever.

Pearl for the practitioner:
Regularly using analgesics 2 or more days per week tends to aggravate chronic headaches, turning intermittent headaches into daily problematic headaches called *analgesic overuse headache*.

Box 8.4 Frequency of Using Prescription Medications That Have Been Linked to Analgesic Overuse Headache (Based on [3])

- Butalbital combinations ≥5 days per month
- Opioids ≥8 days per month
- Triptans ≥10 days per month

Box 8.5 Patient Flyer for Analgesic or Medication Overuse Headaches

What is Medication Overuse Headache?

If you get headaches, taking too many pain medications can actually make your headaches worse. If you get headaches most days and take a pain medication at least 3 days every week, you probably have a worsening of your headaches from the medication or *medication overuse headache*. These headaches used to be called *drug rebound headaches*.

Headache treatments are divided into *acute* and *preventive* therapies. *Acute* therapies treat the headache you have right now.

- Examples of common acute therapies include over-the-counter medications (like Motrin, Excedrin, and Tylenol), prescription pain killers (like Fiorinol, Fioricet, Stadol, and Vicodin), and migraine medications like the triptans (like Imitrex, Maxalt, Zomig, Axert, and Relpax)
- If you are *regularly* taking any individual or a combination of pain or acute migraine pills more than two days a week for more than four to six weeks, you can develop medication overuse headaches

Prevention therapies are treatments you use every day to prevent headaches from happening in the future. People with frequent headaches may take prevention therapies to help with their headaches.

- Examples of prevention therapies include some medications and nonmedication techniques (like relaxation, biofeedback, and stress management). Prevention medications were all originally designed to treat other medical conditions that share some of the same chemicals important for pain and headaches. Types of drugs that are often helpful include some mood elevators, blood pressure medications, and nerve or seizure treatments
- Taking acute medications too often does not help prevent headaches

(continued)

Box 8.5 (continued)

- Taking too many acute medications can actually make it so prevention medications won't work to reduce your headaches until you stop taking the acute therapies

How Can Taking Pain Killers Make My Headaches Worse?

When you take an acute pain or migraine pill every day or nearly every day, your brain changes its chemistry. Chemicals, like serotonin, that are important for sending pain messages get out of balance when you take pain killers too often. This imbalance actually makes you MORE susceptible to getting headaches. And the more pills you keep taking, the worse it gets. In addition, your brain will stop reacting to pain killers it sees too often, so the pills stop working to decrease your pain. When this happens, your brain can also begin to ignore your body's naturally produced pain killers. This causes you to get more headaches and worse headaches. So you'll find that the more pills you take, the less they seem to help. This problem happens with all medications designed to treat a migraine episode. Switching from one pain killer to another doesn't help the problem.

In addition, using acute therapies too often also prevents headache preventive treatments from working. So sometimes the reason nothing seems to help your headaches is because excessive acute medication use is blocking the effectiveness of other therapies.

How Is Medication Overuse Headache Treated?

Everyone says, "Once my headaches are better, I'll be happy to get rid of all of these pills." Unfortunately, your headaches can't get better until the excess medication gets out of your system and your brain has several weeks to rebalance brain chemicals. Your doctor will have you stop or slowly discontinue your daily medication. Over the next month, your doctor may have you take an anti-inflammatory medication (like Aleve) or tramadol (Ultram) for your headaches. These medications are less likely to worsen headaches.

Once you have been off of your over-used medicine, you and your doctor will need to reassess your headache pattern. If you are still having frequent headaches (meaning regularly having troublesome headaches more than 2 or 3 days each week), you will need to start a preventive therapy. If your headaches become infrequent, your doctor may have you go back to using acute

(continued)

Second, this case illustrates the need for ED providers to remain objective and calm when patients become emotional and demanding. Doctors also need to ensure that their own frustration with a busy ED and a demanding patient does not cloud their judgment and cause them to take shortcuts that might result in avoidable diagnostic errors. This chapter provides tips for identifying common sources of errors and suggestions for minimizing errors and conflicts with demanding patients.

Finally, this case shows how engaging in negotiations over the use of inappropriate medications suggests to the patient that this type of bargaining is appropriate. Even when the doctor does not acquiesce to inappropriate patient demands, these encounters teach patients that this type of behavior is acceptable for future ED visits. Using a consistent, caring but firm approach with patients, as will be described below, has been shown to reduce future inappropriate ED visits.

The "Difficult Patient" Encounter

Most healthcare providers identify "difficult" patients as those who are angry, uncooperative, and demanding. In the ED headache patient, this is often the patient who, like Melinda in our case, says, "The *only* thing that ever helps my headache is a shot of Demerol or Dilaudid. And I'm not leaving until I get it!" Although the focus is often placed on the demanding patient, frustrating and nonproductive patient–healthcare provider encounters can usually be attributed to a combination of patient, healthcare provider, and situational factors (Table 8.1) [6].

Table 8.1 Common sources of conflict and suggestions for reactions to defusing them (based on [6])

Factor	Appropriate reaction	Example
A. Patient factors		
Angry, resistant patient	Avoid responding with anger; this can quickly escalate a negative situation. Keep your speech soft and slow to add calm to the situation. Identify what is upsetting or frightening the patient and use reflective statements that show you understand.	Patient complains, "You've kept me waiting for hours. My head is killing me!" Respond, "I can understand why you're upset and I appreciate you being so patient waiting for me. I want to see what I can do to help you."
Manipulative patient	Avoid becoming emotional and reacting out of anger. Don't allow your emotions to escalate. Avoid withholding appropriate treatment just because the patient is unreasonable. Offer and provide reasonable and appropriate treatment and document why the patient's requested therapy was not provided.	Patient threatens, "If you don't give me what I want, I'll sue!" Respond, "This is the appropriate treatment for your condition. The treatment you are requesting is not something that we would use to treat people with your medical condition."
Somatizing patient	Recognize the high level of distress and screen for likely comorbid depression and anxiety.[a]	Patient insists, "I know there's something you've missed. I have to have another test!" Respond, "We've done several examinations to make sure you don't have a serious medical problem. These examinations suggest that you have migraine, which is a real and biological disorder that causes headaches and other problems. The good news is that you can get migraines under control and we're going to help you set up an appointment with a doctor who specializes in this to help you."
Frequent fliers	Don't assume the patient is coming to the ED for narcotics. Ask the patient directly why they frequent the ED for headache management. Screen for comorbid depression and anxiety.[a]	Patients may choose the ED because of problems with insurance, adequate timely post-ED follow-up care was unable to be arranged, or comorbid psychological distress is present. Ensure that an appropriate follow-up plan is in place (see Chap. 9).

(continued)

Table 8.1 (continued)

Factor	Appropriate reaction	Example
B. Physician factors		
Angry, defensive doctor	Recognize high stress level, burnout, or personal issues that might be adding to stress. Excuse yourself to take a short break away from the patient when you sense you're becoming upset; practice relaxation techniques and stretch your muscles to help relieve stress.	Recognize the types of patients/ situations that typically make you upset. Practice deep breathing or other relaxation techniques[b] before starting these encounters. Discuss difficult patient encounters with colleagues, using their expertise and distance from the situation to help identify the best approaches to difficult situations.
Overworked doctor	Recognize the role of fatigue in increasing your emotional response.	Review future schedules to ensure adequate sleep and rest between work shifts.
Dogmatic or arrogant doctor	Recognize that your personal beliefs can cloud your medical judgment. Avoid "judging" the importance or significance of the cause of someone else's distress. Treat all patients equally regardless of gender, race, ethnicity, socioeconomic status, etc. Work hard to minimize stereotypes.	When seeing a headache patient you may think, "Good grief! When I get a headache I certainly don't complain like this! And if she was REALLY in such discomfort she couldn't be as difficult as she is!" Understand that people experience different levels of symptoms with similar medical conditions and tolerance varies among patients.
C. Situational factors		
Language barriers	Talk to patients in language they can understand, avoiding medical terminology and using a translator when necessary.	Use a trained interpreter to help you communicate directly with your patient when possible, rather than speaking to a friend or family member instead of the patient.
Multiple people in the room	Identify who is appropriate to be in the room with the patient and limit the group to that or those individuals. Direct your conversation to the patient rather than others who might be in the room.	Remove others who might be upsetting, controlling, or abusive to the patient or would not be involved in medical decision making.
ED environment	Recognize that excessive stimulation generally aggravates headache complaints and minimize unnecessary light, noise, and activity.	Placing a headache patient in a quiet, dimly lit room away from ED chaos is part of the treatment for primary headaches. For example, turn off the overhead light and direct the exam lamp away from the patient to provide the necessary light to take the history. Use the green filter on the ophthalmoscope to visualize the disc and minimize bright light.

[a] Depression and anxiety screening tools are provided in Chap. 9
[b] Relaxation techniques are provided in Chap. 4

It is important to recognize that "difficult patients" may not be "difficult" people, but individuals under substantial distress due to health concerns [7]. Being a patient in the ED can be frightening and anxiety provoking. Being a patient can be depersonalizing as patients may be asked to reveal intimate details of their personal lives and submit to physical examinations. Recognizing the stress and distress involved with being an ED patient can help make the ED staff more supportive and less likely to react negatively to patient complaints or demands.

Negative staff reactions are generally counterproductive and may aggravate rather than soothe a difficult patient encounter. Physician verbal and nonverbal communication should convey a caring attitude that can help defuse an initially difficult encounter:

- Stay calm, assured, and avoid raising your voice;
- Sit down while the patient provides a history;
- Retain good eye contact;
- Avoid completing other work while the patient is talking;
- Show you're an active listener by reflecting statements back to the patient;
- Always use effective communication strategies (Table 8.2) [8].

> **Pearl for the practitioner:**
> *Reflective listening* involves paraphrasing what your patient tells you to make sure the meaning is clear when you say it in your own words. Reflective listening is important for effective communication and to show patients that you are engaged or interested in what they are saying. An example would be, "So let me get this straight, you were camping in northwest Wisconsin about 3 weeks before the headaches worsened? Is that correct?"

Table 8.2 Effective communication strategies (based on [8])

Communication strategy	Example
Ask–tell–ask communication	*Ask* patients to explain concerns in their own words: "*What are you most concerned about?*"
	Tell patients important information (e.g., diagnosis and treatment recommendations) using easy-to-understand language: "*Based on my examination today, the cause of your head pain is likely to be migraine. A CT scan is not usually necessary when your symptoms suggest a migraine.*"
	Ask patients to rephrase your message using their own words to ensure effective communication: "*To let me know that you understood what I told you, tell me in your own words what you heard me say is causing your head pain.*"
Open-ended questions	Limit questions to which patients can provide simply a "yes" or "no" response. Ask "*What does your head feel like*" instead of "*Is the pain throbbing?*"

Recognizing Drug-Seeking Behavior

According to the 2007–2008 National Survey on Drug Use and Health, pain reliev-
ers are the second most common illicit drug of abuse after marijuana [9]. Over the
last two decades, there has been a marked increase in the use of opioids for the treatment of chronic nonmalignant pain, with an unfortunate increase in the prevalence
of opioid abuse (Box 8.6) [10]. Consequently, healthcare providers, including ED
staff, will likely be confronted with patients feigning or exaggerating illness to

---

Box 8.6 Opioid Abuse Statistics (Based on [10])

- The Partnership for a Drug-Free America survey of teens found that

  - 61% of teens agree that prescription drugs are easier to get than illegal
    street drugs
  - 41% believe prescription and over-the-counter drugs with abuse poten-
    tial are less dangerous than street drugs
  - 20% have abused prescription drugs to get high

- Nearly 40% of all poisoning deaths in 2006 were caused by opioids

  - Fatal opioid poisonings rose from 4,000 in 1999 to 13,800 deaths in 2006

Box 8.7 Red Flags for Drug-Seeking Behavior (Based on [14])

- The patient is "allergic" to multiple common nonopioid headache
  medications
- The patient is a frequent flier in the ED who usually requests opioids
- The patient has not completed or continued follow-up with an outpatient
  headache provider
- The patient requests specific pain medications ("The only thing that ever
  works for me is Demerol")
- Reported pain severity seems to conflict with observed behavior (e.g., the
  patient reports pain as "12" on a severity scale from 1 to 10, but is pleas-
  antly chatting with friends who accompanied her to the ED)
- The patient displays manipulative behavior
- The patient has a history of losing prescriptions, running out of the medication before it should be gone, and/or using other people's medications
- The patient often presents after hours, is in a hurry, and is from "out of
  town"

Box 8.8 Six Characteristics Linked to Opioid Seeking in the ED (Based on [15])

- Using an alias
- Requesting to be seen by specific or different doctor
- Noncompliance with primary care appointments
- Reporting lost, stolen, or damaged medications
- Displaying threatening or abusive behavior when a prescription is denied
- Physician uneasiness over prescribing a controlled substance

receive drugs of abuse. It is estimated that an ED treating 75,000 patients annually can expect up to 262 monthly visits from patients seeking drugs [11].

Surveys report comorbid substance abuse in up to one in three ED visits [12, 13]. Many kits are available that can quickly test for drugs of abuse. Obtaining a rapid turn-around urine drug screen for possible illicit drug use early in the visit can provide valuable information to the treating clinician. The ED can also be an excellent venue for initiating referrals for substance abuse evaluation and treatment among patients suspected of having abuse problems (Boxes 8.7 and 8.8) [11, 14, 15].

Approaching the Patient Who Insists on Inappropriate Treatment

Headache patients who insist on a specific therapy may do so for several reasons. They may have had previous good success with that treatment; they may have heard about the effectiveness of this treatment from others; or they may be seeking medication for other purposes, e.g., opioids for recreational use. Providing patients with clear messages and explanations can help reduce inappropriate demands. It is important to clearly define early on in the encounter what the provider will and will not do to treat the headache pain. It is important to remember that physicians are under no obligation to provide specific options or prescribe medications that they are not comfortable prescribing. In cases where patients are requesting a specific medication that you would not feel comfortable providing, be clear that you do not provide this therapy and provide reasons for not prescribing (e.g., Demerol may not be prescribed because of too many side effects, the risk for accumulation of dangerous metabolites, and limited efficacy for headache pain).

Consistently implementing specific strategies to reduce inappropriate ED visits was shown to be successful in a pilot study of problem patients [16]. In this study, 24 patients identified as frequently making ED visits for chronic conditions and displaying drug seeking or abusive behavior were treated with the following restrictions:

- Prescriptions for opioids and benzodiazepines were not provided;
- Patients were referred to a primary care physician and appropriate additional services;

- Attention-seeking behaviors were not rewarded by "fast-tracking" patients into an examination room rather than allowing patients to disrupt the waiting room;
- Patients were given supportive counseling.

The number of ED visits decreased from 616 visits during the 12 months before implementing these strategies to 175 during the year after changing the ED approach. Having a clear approach that was understood and consistently applied by the ED staff were the keys to the success of this program.

Patients need to understand that you will not get involved in a treatment negotiation. One useful approach is to use the acronym BOSS to frame the visit:

- B for boundaries
- O for options
- S for scripting responses
- S for sincerity

Boundaries

Boundaries should be established early in the patient encounter, clarifying what the provider is and is not willing to do (Table 8.3). By explicitly outlining the recommended

Table 8.3 Setting boundaries for therapeutic options

What the patient is thinking	When I was here before, they gave me Demerol for my headache. That's what I want again.
What the patient says	Unfortunately, I am allergic to most headache medications. Last time, they gave me something that started with a "D" that worked really well.
Example of poor boundary setting	
What the doctor is thinking	Her again?! Wasn't she just here yesterday for a shot of Demerol? Luckily my shift ends in 15 min and I can pass her on to the next guy. He can argue with her about the Demerol.
What the doctor says	Let me go look up your records and see if I can find what worked for you before.
Example of good boundary setting	
What the doctor is thinking	Her again?! Wasn't she just here yesterday for a shot of Demerol? I need to make it clear that she won't be getting this again.
What the doctor says	Yesterday, you were given a shot of Demerol. Since you're back here today, that medication is not effective in getting rid of your migraine. Now that we know that Demerol is not effective for you, we can avoid giving you Demerol or other opioid medications for your headaches. We will give you a different type of treatment today and make sure you get an appointment with a headache doctor who will manage your headaches.

treatment approach, the eventual "test of wills" that can occur ("I am not going to leave until I get my Demerol" vs. "There is no way that I am going to give in this time") can be avoided or minimized. Many times, when a drug-seeking patient knows from the start that they will not be given narcotics, they realize that they are wasting their time and leave.

Options

As described in Chap. 4, there is a broad assortment of possible effective treatments for common primary headaches, like migraine, seen in the ED. Utilizing a full range of possible treatments provides a number of potential nonopioid treatment options that will usually include therapies tolerated by patients reporting numerous medication sensitivities and allergies.

Scripting Responses

Having a clear, concise way to consistently explain the headache treatment approach offered to an individual patient and the rationale behind these recommendations can be extremely useful in the ED. Anticipating common concerns or issues that patients may have and utilizing practiced responses can improve the confidence the practitioner displays to the patient and help avoid confrontations (Table 8.4).

Sincerity

While some headache patients in the ED may be drug seeking, most patients are in the ED because they are having problematic headaches and they are sincerely looking for an evaluation and headache relief. Treating all patients with respect goes a long way toward defusing potentially unpleasant encounters. It is important to be compassionate when refusing to provide an inappropriate therapy that a patient may be requesting and clearly stating that the requested medication is considered to be inappropriate and may be potentially harmful for the patient [11]. The healthcare provider's attitude and demeanor should help the patient see that the provider is working in the patient's best interest, even when the provider is not dispensing therapy that might have been expected or requested by the patient.

> ***Pearl for the practitioner:***
> Be the **BOSS** when confronting patients making unreasonable requests:
>
> - Set appropriate **B**oundaries to let patients know early on what you are and are not willing to prescribe
> - Utilize a range of treatment **O**ptions so you have a full armamentarium to use in patients who report multiple drug sensitivities and allergies
> - **S**cript responses to common concerns in advance to improve your confidence in delivering clear answers to typical patient concerns
> - Show patients your **S**incerity by treating them with respect, fully addressing their concerns, and letting them know you won't provide treatment that you think may cause harm over either the short- or long-term

Table 8.4 Common patient concerns and possible ED staff responses

Patient concern	Provider response
Why can't I just have my Demerol?	There are many options used to treat headache pain. The best approach is to treat the underlying cause by using headache-specific medications. Medications like Demerol are not helpful for chronic headaches for several reasons. Demerol is very short acting, so the effect wears off quickly so most people are at risk for having their headache come back. Taking Demerol too often can also make your headache worse. This can cause what's called *analgesic overuse headaches*. Demerol can change the way the brain perceives pain, so your next headache can seem even worse and be more difficult to treat. Demerol is also addictive.
That stuff never works	I realize that you may have not had good results in the past with medications other than Demerol. I would like to try a variety of medications from different classes that treat the headache from different angles. I will also give you instructions on what you need to do while you're treating your headache and combining these techniques with other treatments will make those other treatment more effective.
How do you know that I don't have a brain tumor?	While it is extremely difficult to rule out a brain tumor with 100% accuracy, your symptoms and my exam today point to a more common type of headache. If the headache doesn't respond to the treatments that I prescribe or if the symptoms change, you can work with your primary care doctor to look into this further.
Why don't you think that I need a MRI?	An MRI scan can be very helpful in finding certain problems in the brain. Your headaches are consistent with migraines, which don't show up on an MRI scan. Migraine is a real problem that can cause severe headaches and other symptoms. Migraine is caused by a chemical imbalance that can't be detected with x-rays or blood tests.
The guy who I saw last week gave me 20 Vicodin to take home.	While different doctors have different approaches to treating pain, the best approach in my opinion is not to use narcotics like Vicodin. I do not use narcotic medications for headache pain because they are generally ineffective in treating headache symptoms, have high addiction potential, and can actually make the headache pain worse and more difficult to treat. There are other more effective headache medications.

Reducing the Risk of Litigation

Focusing on effective communication is essential for establishing a patient–physician relationship that includes trust and respect. In addition, recognizing and eliminating common errors in the thought process involved in decision making can help avoid typical diagnostic pitfalls and improve diagnostic accuracy.

Communicating to Reduce Litigation Risk

Research shows that patients often pursue litigation because they wanted greater communication and honesty from their healthcare providers, recognition of the injury they received, and assurances that lessons would be learned from their experience [17]. Attending to achieving effective communication is linked to a reduced risk for malpractice claims in primary care (Table 8.5) [18]. Interestingly, this research found less of a link between the *content* of a conversation than the *process* of communication and *tone* of the visit for predicting malpractice suits. A Canadian survey likewise identified poor communication as a predictor of complaints against physicians, with the most commonly reported reason for the complaint being a problem with physician attitude or communication (57% of all complaints) [19]. While these studies did not specifically evaluate ED patients, the same principles of good communication are important in the ED and will likely similarly reduce a patient's likelihood of pursuing complaints.

> ***Pearl for the practitioner:***
> Poor communication is an important predictor of future malpractice litigation.

Table 8.5 Communication techniques linked to reduced malpractice risk (based on [18])

Technique	Example
Explaining what the patient should expect throughout the visit	"First, I'm going to talk to you about your headaches and then do an examination. Then we'll decide if any tests are needed to help make the diagnosis. Then we'll have time to talk about how to treat your headache and other concerns you might have."
Letting patients know their opinions matter	"Tell me more about that concern." "What do you think is causing your head pain?" "What have you heard about different migraine treatments?"
Showing warmth, friendliness, and humor	Approaching patients with an open, friendly attitude helps patients feel their doctor's warmth and makes patients want to feel personally connected to the doctor. Make certain that humor is appropriate for the individual situation.

Recognizing Common Diagnostic and Judgment Errors

Psychologists typically describe physician decision making as a two-step process using the Dual Process Theory [20]. According to this model, the first step involves intuitive, automatic decisions. These decisions are then moderated by the second step that includes analytical reasoning. Doctors need to use both of these steps to improve their diagnostic accuracy. Excessive reliance on initial thoughts in step one can result in a failure to consider diagnoses that are not commonly seen in an individual's personal practice. Failure to adjust current practice to incorporate well-developed clinical guidelines is another example of excessive dependence on step one decision making. Often, however, initial impressions are correct and excessive reliance on step two can leave doctors endlessly considering additional remote possibilities and constantly second guessing themselves.

Cognitive Errors

A survey of the cases of diagnostic error for 100 retrospectively reviewed internal medicine cases identified cognitive errors (problems with information, data collection, or data synthesis) as the most common cause of error, contributing to errors in 74% of cases [21]. Interestingly, cognitive errors occurred more commonly than technical failures/organizational flaws or errors related to uncooperative or deceptive patients or unusual disease presentations. Cognitive errors were divided into those caused by errors in:

- Information processing – 50% of all instances of cognitive errors;
- Information verification – 33%;
- Data gathering – 14%;
- Knowledge – 3%.

The most common individual error was termed *premature closure*, described as a tendency to stop considering other likely diagnostic possibilities too soon in the diagnostic process. Incomplete history and physical examination data, bias toward a single diagnosis, and failure to include the correct diagnosis among the considered choices all contribute to premature closure errors. While this study did not involve an evaluation of ED patients, these same principles can be applied to ED diagnosis (see Table 8.6 for examples of cognitive errors that might occur with the ED headache patient present in Case 1).

> *Pearl for the practitioner:*
> Premature closure, a tendency to limit diagnostic possibilities too soon during an evaluation, is one of the most common causes of diagnostic errors.

Table 8.6 Examples of common cognitive errors

Type of error	Description	Example from Case 1
Context errors	Only a limited number of diagnostic possibilities are considered	The patient has a history of migraine and is likely drug seeking. Physician did not fully examine the patient and missed the bull's eye rash on her back. Physician dismissed the fact that she had a low grade fever for the week prior to the ED visit.
Availability errors	Diagnostic choice is limited to those conditions with which one is most familiar or which one considers to be the most common	Migraine is far more common than headaches related to Lyme disease, which was not considered.
Premature closure errors	Once a reasonable solution is identified, all other possibilities are not fully considered	Since the patient had a history of migraine headache and appeared to be drug seeking, the physician failed to consider the possibility of less common causes of headaches such as Lyme disease.

The importance of cognitive errors in ED malpractice claims is supported by a review of 79 claims involving a missed diagnosis in the ED that harmed a patient [22]. In this survey, the leading factors contributing to missed diagnoses were cognitive factors (96% of cases). The most common individual areas of error were failure to order an appropriate test (58%), failure to obtain an adequate history or physical examination (42%), incorrect test interpretation (37%), and failure to request consultation (33%).

Signal-to-Noise Errors

Signal-to-noise errors refer to the need to separate important clinical information from the wealth of background noise of data collected from a patient's history and examination [20]. This can be particularly difficult when presentations of benign and life-threatening diagnoses overlap (e.g., migraine and subarachnoid hemorrhage).

Healthcare provider decisions may also be inappropriately affected by factors that are not related to the likelihood of one diagnosis over another, such as race, ethnicity, and gender. Although these factors may be important for some diagnoses, they often are extraneous to appropriate care and decisions. In a disturbing recent study, race/ethnicity appeared to be linked to likelihood of obtaining computed tomography (CT) imaging in 155 patients with headache seen in the ED [23]. Most patients in this sample were African-American (41%) or Hispanic (33%), with 17% white and 9% other. A CT scan was ordered for 57 patients (37%), with an abnormal result obtained in 6 cases (11%). Abnormalities included hematoma, brain mass, sinusitis, and infarct, none of which were considered to be acutely life threatening. Patients were appropriately more likely to have received a CT when they had a higher predicted severity based on the Emergency Severity Index (ESI) [24] (for patients with ESI $\leq$ 3, odds ratio = 5.11; 95% CI 1.53–17.12; $P < 0.01$). Patients were disturbingly less likely to have received a head CT if they were African-American (odds ratio = 0.21; 95% confidence interval [CI] −0.09– 0.52; $P < 0.01$). Outcome data were not provided to determine whether the presence of abnormalities was higher among certain groups or whether long-term evaluations confirmed that imaging studies were or were not indicated among those patients not receiving an imaging study. These data, however, do highlight the need to ensure that decisions for pursuing testing are based on clinically relevant characteristics to make certain that all patients are receiving optimal care.

Attitude Errors

Overconfidence has also been linked to diagnostic errors [25, 26]. Overconfidence may result in failure to consider other diagnosis, failure to consult available resources, and failure to obtain appropriate specialty consultation.

Strategies for Reducing Common Errors

Experts encourage the use of metacognition (defined as "thinking about thinking") to help reduce common diagnostic errors [27]. Metacognition requires an awareness of limitations in decision making and memory, an ability to step back and see that there may be broader possibilities to a diagnosis than initially identified, and a willingness to critique one's decision-making process. It is also important to understand common pitfalls in the decision-making process, such as the errors listed above, and recognize how these errors might occur in the ED. Specific strategies for reducing errors are given in Box 8.9 [28].

Box 8.9 Strategies for Reducing Common Errors (Based on [27])

- Recognize the role of cognitive, signal-to-noise, and attitude errors
- Consider a range of alternative diagnoses
- After initial diagnosis has been established, step back and evaluate the decision-making process for possible errors
- Decrease reliance on memory by using available resources, algorithms, practice guidelines, etc
- Obtain and utilize all available information
- Allow adequate time for decision making
- Participate in simulation training exercises to help identify common errors when addressing typical clinical scenarios
- Become accountable for your decisions by following up to verify accuracy and review cases where errors have been identified. Encourage feedback from others about subsequent patient outcome to assist this process. Consider routine independent review of cases in your department by colleagues to promote discussions of best practices

Box 8.10 Summary Tips on Avoiding Common Pitfalls in Communication and Diagnosis in the ED

- Keep an open mind – don't jump to conclusions and avoid limiting your assessment and diagnosis based on irrelevant patient factors, including patient emotional responses
- Make communicating with the patient a top priority

  - Be an active listener
  - Listen without interrupting
  - Use open-ended questions and reflect statements back to patients to verify good understanding
  - Uses Ask–Tell–Ask techniques to ensure correct information is communicated

- Remember body language is an important communication tool. If you're feeling stressed and emotional, take a mini-break to compose yourself so you can present your best, calm, caring, interested self to the patient
- Don't take short cuts – use a standard approach for evaluating patients to avoid missing important clues in the history or examination
- Document clearly – including what your thought processes were, how a diagnosis was reached, and why specific therapies were recommended. When patients have requested a therapy that is not being offered, be sure to document why this therapy was not appropriate/not prescribed

Box 8.10 (continued)

- Obtain written consent for all procedures – use reflective statements when talking to patients to make sure you understand and address their concerns
- Provide the patient with written instructions about test results, medications given during the visit, symptoms that should prompt a return visit, interim medications, and follow-up (available in Chap. 9)
- Don't forget to ask all females about contraception and possible risk for pregnancy. Ask new mothers whether they might be nursing to help guide therapy choices
- Maintain a current knowledge base of risk factors for drug seeking, pharmacokinetics of common pain medications, drug interactions, and laws regarding scheduled medications
- Remember to warn patients about avoiding decision making and activities like driving when prescribing therapies with cognitive effects. Similarly, provide written instructions on restrictions after minor head injury, when appropriate (available in Chap. 3)
- When possible, consult with the patient's primary care or headache-treating provider
- Don't hesitate to ask for a consult for difficult cases or cases where diagnosis or treatment selection is unclear or problematic

Understanding Local Malpractice Laws

While most states have similar legal requirements for treating clinicians, physicians must understand the specific requirements that apply to the state where they are practicing. Reviewing how courts instruct jurors to make their decisions in medical malpractice cases can also be helpful.

General guidelines that typically apply to malpractice cases are described below:

- Physicians generally are not judged on the outcome, but rather whether the standards of care for their specialty were met. Unfortunately, physicians may not agree on the standard of care for many conditions and there can be >1 standard of care or approach to individual problems. Expert testimony is often used to define the standard of care in court.
- If a physician relies on the "recognized method of treatment" defense, he/she is obligated to have told the patient that >1 recognized method of care was available as part of the informed consent process.
- Informed consent is becoming a very important malpractice strategy for patients' attorneys. One of the reasons that informed consent is gaining popularity is that this defense is not based on the standards of care that a *reasonable physician* would follow, but rather what a *reasonable patient* would want to know. In

many states, expert testimony is not required to evaluate the completeness of informed consent; instead, testimony can be used to determine if the physician provided all of the reasonable options that a reasonable patient would want to know. There have been cases where the physician was found not guilty on the basis of whether he provided care that met the standard of care in the community, but was found guilty on the grounds that he did not provide adequate informed consent.

• Physicians need to know how their state defines malpractice.

Case 2

An ED physician was successfully sued for treating a 35-year-old patient presenting to the ED with a "usual headache." Because there was no indication of trauma, infection, or another secondary cause for the headache, imaging studies were not performed. The patient was treated, discharged, and suffered a stroke several days later. Because the patient had not been informed specialty imaging studies and neurologic consultation were not available at the hospital where he had been treated, he successfully sued based on insufficient informed consent for failure to discuss options. The physician might have avoided this litigation by having informed the patient that his examination did not warrant an imaging study during the ED visit, but that he might need to be scheduled for imaging or a neurological consultation should symptoms persist or worsen.

Additional Resources

• *Avoiding Common Errors in the Emergency Department* by Amal Mattu et al., 2010.
• *Emergency Medicine: Avoiding the Pitfalls and Improving the Outcomes* by Amal Mattu and Deepi Goyal, 2007.
• *Field Guide to the Difficult Patient Interview* by Fredric W. Platt and Geoffrey H. Gordon, 2004.

Summary

• ED physicians ranked fifth in frequency of malpractice claims. However, nearly half of all ED physicians will be sued at some point in their careers. Much can be done to minimize the risk of litigation.
• Using effective communication techniques, being cognizant of common diagnostic pitfalls, and understanding the laws of the state in which an ED is located can significantly reduce the risk of litigation.

- The acronym BOSS can help frame the ED visit by setting *B*oundaries, considering a host of effective *O*ptions, *S*cripting responses to common questions, and being *S*incere in your approach to the patient.
- Prematurely discontinuing consideration of alternative diagnostic options is one of the most common thought process errors during diagnosis setting.
- Metacognition strategies analyzing the thought process and critiquing decision making can help identify and reduce diagnostic errors.
- Understanding how your state defines malpractice is important.
- ED providers should clearly understand the concept of informed consent as it has become a common strategy used in litigation for malpractice attorneys.

References

1. Kane CK. Medical liability claim frequency: a 2007–2008 snapshot of physicians. AMA Center for Economics and Health Policy Research, Aug 2010. http://www.ama-assn.org/ama1/pub/upload/mm/363/prp-201001-claim-freq.pdf. Accessed Nov 2010.
2. Brown TW, McCarthy ML, Kelen GD, Levy F. An epidemiologic study of closed emergency department malpractice claims in a national database of physician malpractice insurers. Acad Emerg Med. 2010;17:553–60.
3. Bigal ME, Serrano D, Buse D, et al. Acute migraine medications and evolution from episodic to chronic migraine: a longitudinal population-based study. Headache. 2008;48:1157–68.
4. Tepper SJ, Tepper DE. Breaking the cycle of medication overuse headache. Cleveland Clinic J Med. 2010;77:236–42.
5. Supornsilpchai W, le Grand SM, Srikiatkhaachorn A. Involvement of pro-nociceptive 5-HT2A receptor in the pathogenesis of medication-overuse headache. Headache. 2010;50:185–97.
6. Hull SK, Broquet K. How to manage difficult patient encounters. Fam Pract Manage. 2007;14: 30–4.
7. Baum N. Dealing with difficult patients. J Med Pract Manage. 2009;25:33–6.
8. Buse DC, Rupnow MT, Lipton RB. Assessing and managing all aspects of migraine: migraine attacks, migraine-related functional impairment, common comorbidities, and quality of life. Mayo Clin Proc. 2009;84:422–35.
9. US Department of Health and Human Services SAMHSA website http://www.oas.samhsa.gov/. Accessed October 2010.
10. Saper JR, Lake AE, Bain PA, et al. A practice guide for continuous opioid therapy for refractory daily headache: patient selection, physician requirements, and treatment monitoring. Headache. 2010;50:1175–93.
11. Hansen GR. The drug-seeking patient in the emergency room. Emerg Med Clin N Am. 2005;23:349–65.
12. Rockett IR, Putnam SL, Jioa H, Smith GS. Assessing substance abuse treatment need: a statewide hospital emergency department study. Ann Emerg Med. 2003;41:802–13.
13. D-Onofrio G, Degutis LC. Integrating Project ASSERT: a screening, intervention, and referral to treatment program for unhealthy alcohol and drug use in to an urban emergency department. Acad Emerg Med. 2010;17:903–11.
14. Longo LP, Parran T, Johnson B, Kinsey W. Addiction: part II. Identification and management of the drug-seeking patients. Am Fam Physician. 2000;61:2401–8.
15. Chan L, Winegard B. Attributes and behaviors associated with opioid seeking in the emergency department. J Opioid Manage. 2007;3:244–8.
16. Pope D, Fernandes CB, Bouthillette F, Etherington J. Frequent users of the emergency department: a program to improve care and reduce visits. Can Med Assoc J. 2000;162:1017–20.

17. Vincent C, Phillips A, Young M. Why do people sue doctors? A study of patients and relatives taking legal action. Lancet. 1999;343:1609–13.
18. Levinson W, Roter DL, Mullooly JP, Dull VT, Frankel R. Physician–patient communication. The relationship with malpractice claims among primary care physicians and surgeons. JAMA. 1997;227:553–9.
19. Tamblyn R, Abrahamowicz M, Dauphinee D, et al. Physician scores on a national clinical skills examination as predictors of complaints to medical regulatory authorities. JAMA. 2007;298:993–1001.
20. Croskerry P. Context is everything or how could I have been that stupid? Healthc Q. 2009;12:e171–7.
21. Graber ML, Franklin N, Gordon R. Diagnostic error in internal medicine. Arch Intern Med. 2005;165:1493–9.
22. Kachalia A, Gandhi TK, Puopolo AL, et al. Missed and delayed diagnoses in the emergency department: a study of closed malpractice claims from 4 liability insurers. Ann Emerg Med. 2007;49:196–205.
23. Harris B, Hwang U, Lee WS, Richardson LD. Disparities in use of computed tomography for patients presenting with headache. Am J Emerg Med. 2009;27:333–6.
24. Elshove-Bolk J, Mencl F, van Rijwijck BF, et al. Validation of the Emergency Severity Index (ESI) in self-referred patients in a European emergency department. Emerg Med J. 2007;24:170–4.
25. Berner ES, Graber ML. Overconfidence as a cause of diagnostic error in medicine. Am J Med. 2008;121:S2–23.
26. Norman GR, Eva KW. Diagnostic and clinical reasoning. Med Educ. 2010;44:94–100.
27. Croskerry P. Cognitive forcing strategies in clinical decisionmaking. Ann Emerg Med. 2003;41:110–20.
28. Croskerry P. The importance of cognitive errors in diagnosis and strategies to minimize them. Acad Med. 2003;78:775–80.
29. Zeeberg P, Olesen J, Jensen R. Discontinuation of medication overuse in headache patients: recovery of therapeutic responsiveness. Cephalalgia. 2006;26:1192–8.
30. Rapoport AM, Weeks RE, Sheftell FD, Baskin SM, Verdi J. The "analgesic washout period": a critical variable in the evaluation of treatment efficacy. Neurology. 1986;36 Suppl 1:100–1.

Chapter 9
After the ED: Arranging Post-ED
Follow-up Care

Key Chapter Points

- Patients treated in the ED for acute headache have a high rate of return visits.
- The reasons for the high rate of return visits may include recurrence of severe headache pain, lack of an effective interim treatment plan and medications, and an inability to be seen by a headache-interested provider in a timely manner.
- Return visits can be reduced by effectively treating headache pain and nausea in the ED, providing the patient with a clear, written interim treatment strategy, providing prescriptions for effective medications that can be used in the interim, and facilitating timely follow up with a headache-interested provider.

Keywords Follow up • Recurrence • Return visit

> **Case**
>
> "I always come to the Emergency Department for my headaches. I know some of the doctors and nurses here probably think I'm just coming in for drugs, but it really seems to help my headache when I come to the Emergency Department. My regular doctor doesn't like to hear about my headaches so it's easier to come here. I don't know why they always look so surprised when I come back. I always tell them I get a bad migraine about every other week. And when I do, I come right back to Emergency!"

Most nontraumatic headaches seen in the emergency department (ED) are recurrent, primary headaches. Consequently, many patients, like in our case, may return to the ED for continued headache treatment. A survey of patients receiving ED treatment for a chief complaint of headache reported that only 22% were pain-free on discharge, with mild pain in 42% and moderate to severe pain in the remainder (Fig. 9.1) [1].

D.A. Marcus and P.A. Bain, *Practical Assessment and Treatment of the Patient*   193
with Headaches in the Emergency Department and Urgent Care Clinic,
DOI 10.1007/978-1-4614-0002-8_9, © Springer Science+Business Media, LLC 2011

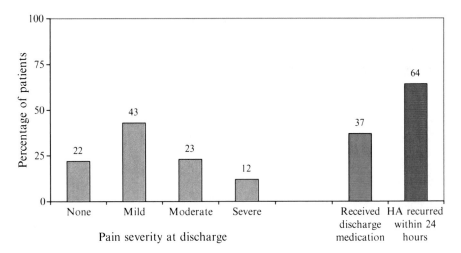

Fig. 9.1   Post-ED headache treatment (based on [1]). *HA* headache

Discharge medications were provided to only 37% of patients. Migraine was the most common diagnosis, which would typically be expected to recur. Headache returned within 24 h in two of three patients. Unfortunately, only 41% of patients were advised to arrange follow-up with a physician for headache management. Having a consistent, detailed discharge plan including an interim treatment strategy, prescriptions for a small amount of effective medications to treat pain and nausea until the patient can be seen in outpatient follow-up, and follow-up arrangements to see a headache-interested provider can reduce inappropriate return visits for acute headache.

> **Pearl for the practitioner:**
> Expect headaches to recur in most patients presenting to the ED with primary headache. Patients will, therefore, need clear and, ideally, written postdischarge treatment recommendations, interim medications, and plans for follow-up.

Patients discharged with a diagnosis of primary headache should be provided with both nonmedication instructions and medications that they can administer at home rather than waiting for headache severity and disability to increase, which may precipitate a repeat ED visit:

- Provide interim nonmedication and medication instructions;
- Offer a limited supply of appropriate interim medications;
- Give the patient clear, written information about their diagnosis, their ED visit, and what to do about residual or recurring headaches;
- Arrange for follow-up with a headache-interested outpatient provider.

Addressing each of these areas is essential for good headache management to minimize unnecessary repeat ED visits.

Provide Interim Care

Patients treated in the ED often continue to report headaches. In one study of patients treated in the ED for headache, moderate to severe headache continued to be reported 24 h after discharge in 31% of patients with migraine and 19% with tension-type headache [2]. Furthermore, patients with primary headaches successfully treated in the ED typically experience a recurrence of their headaches after discharge. In one study, follow-up phone interviews were conducted for 383 patients 48 h after they had been treated with parenteral medications in the ED for a primary headache and discharged to home [3]. For interim migraine treatment therapy, patients were randomly provided with naproxen 500 mg or sumatriptan 100 mg capsules to use if their headaches returned. Headache recurred within 48 h of ED treatment for 73% of patients, with a moderate or severe headache endorsed by half. Headache was reduced to mild or no headache in 72% treated with naproxen and 73% treated with sumatriptan. This study highlights two major points of ED headache treatment:

1. Patients treated for primary headache in the ED will usually have their headaches return within 2 days of discharge.
2. Providing patients with effective primary headache outpatient treatment can successfully treat recurring headaches and prevent unnecessary return to the ED.

Provide Written Instructions for Effective Interim Headache Treatment

Failure to provide a clear postdischarge plan for persistent or recurrent headache may result in unnecessary repeat ED visits. Patients are often groggy after headache treatment (which may also be part of the postdrome phase of a migraine) and may not be able to accurately understand or remember follow-up recommendations. Communicating post-ED treatment recommendations can be substantially enhanced by providing clear, easy-to-understand, written after-care instructions. Including the patient's family or significant support persons in the discharge discussion with the patient can additionally help reduce confusion and improve compliance. The patient should also be encouraged to take these instructions to their appointment with their primary care or other headache-interested provider to facilitate communication. In addition, providing a contact person that the patient can call between ED discharge and follow-up appointments can minimize unnecessary return visits for treatment clarification by:

- Reducing patient anxiety about what to do if headaches worsen;
- Reinforcing appropriate strategies for managing persistent or recurring headaches;
- Offering advice for recurring headaches to reduce unnecessary ED visits for chronic primary headache.

Interim instructions should include both medication and nondrug treatment options that the patient can use to treat their headaches. Options for interim instructions are provided in Boxes 9.1 and 9.2. Instructions sheets on relaxation techniques and exercises provided in Chap. 4 can also be provided.

Rehydration is an important part of acute ED treatment for headache. Encouraging ongoing outpatient hydration can help reduce headache recurrence. In an interesting case study, a computer engineer with migraine successfully reduced headache activity and reliance on medication by programming an electronic prompt to remind him several times throughout the day to drink extra water [4]. Using this system, his daily free water intake improved from about 100 to 1,500 mL/day and headache activity was reduced by half. Medication use was also cut in half. A pilot study likewise showed that patients instructed to increase water intake by 1.5 L daily over 12 weeks experienced improved headaches [5]. Patients assigned to the increased water intake group actually increased water intake by about 1 L daily. The amount of time patients experienced headaches decreased by 38% in the group increasing their fluid intake compared with a 2% increase in headache time for controls. Average headache severity was reduced 13% among fluid drinkers vs. a 28% worsening in controls. A practical strategy is to recommend that a migraine patient use a 1-L bottle for water, drinking at least two bottles of water daily.

Box 9.1 ED Discharge Summary Sheet – Acute Headache

_____(patient name) were seen in the ED on ____/____/_____ for an acute headache.
The discharge diagnosis was: □ Migraine □ _____
Treatment received in the ED included:

□ Hydration
□ Intravenous medications:_____
□ Procedure:_____
□ Other: _____

Tests ordered and results included:

□ Radiographic study:_____
□ Spinal fluid analysis: _____
□ Blood tests:_____
□ Other:_____

Please make a follow-up visit within the next 2 weeks (call to make appointment on the next business day) with:

□ Your primary care provider:_____
□ Your neurologist/headache specialist:_____
□ Another healthcare provider:_____

(continued)

Box 9.1 (continued)

Treatment strategy for your headaches to use between now and when you see your provider:

◻ Nondrug options: relaxation techniques, exercise, sleep, hydration, other____
◻ Nausea medication:

  ○ Ondansetron _____
  ○ Metoclopramide _____
  ○ Prochlorperazine _____

◻ Pain medication:

  ○ Excedrin _____
  ○ Ibuprofen _____
  ○ Naproxen _____
  ○ Sumatriptan _____
  ○ Other:_____

When should I come back to the Emergency Department?

Return to the Emergency Department if you develop slurred speech, excessive sleepiness (it is difficult to wake you up), unsteady walking, weakness of an arm or a leg, or uncontrolled vomiting, or if you develop other new or uncontrollable problems.

If you have questions about your headache or headache therapy before your appointment with your doctor, please call _____.

Box 9.2 Effective Strategies for Reducing Chronic Headaches

1. *Practice relaxation techniques*

   Relaxation techniques are specific skills you learn to turn off pain centers and turn on calming centers in your brain. When you are first learning these skills, you will need to practice for about 15–20 min a couple of times each day. Once you have learned these skills, you can use them when you start feeling an increase in headaches.

   Find additional relaxation and stress management skills at these websites:

   • American Chronic Pain Association 5-min relaxation exercise at http://www.theacpa.org. Enter the word "relaxation" in the search box of the "Resource Finder" and select the resource "Relaxation Guide."
   • Dean Health System resource on stress management at http://www.deancare.com//stress.
   • HelpGuide relaxation tips at http://www.helpguide.org. Use the search word "relaxation."
   • LoveToKnow provides a list of stress reduction resources at http://stress.lovetoknow.com, including downloadable relaxation guides at the

(continued)

Box 9.2 (continued)

"Free Guided Relaxation" link on under the list of "Stress Management Techniques."

2. *Exercise everyday*

Daily aerobic exercise has been proven to help reduce headache activity. Plan to walk a total of 150 min per week. You can do this by exercising for 10 min, three times a day, 5 days each week. Or you can do longer exercise sessions on some days. Try to do some aerobic exercise at least 5 days each week. Examples of effective exercise are walking, walking your dog, bicycling, and swimming. If you have been very inactive or have health problems, talk to your doctor about the way to start an exercise program.

You should also add daily stretches to your exercise routine. Practice neck exercises to help keep headaches away and try these when head pain begins.

3. *Get enough sleep*

Research proves that people get more headaches when they sleep too little or sleep too much. Try to get between 7 and 8 h of sleep each night. Set up and stick to a regular sleeping routine, so you're going to bed and getting up around the same times each day. Avoid caffeine and alcohol before going to bed.

4. *Get enough to drink*

Most people don't get enough to drink. You should try to drink about ten 8-ounce glasses of water each day. Drink extra water before and after exercise. Research shows that headache activity decreases when people get enough daily water. Keep a 1-L bottle filled with water to drink from throughout the day, making sure you drink about two bottles of water daily.

5. *Avoid nicotine*

Smoking or using other nicotine products causes changes in your brain's pain chemicals that can actually increase your sensitivity to pain. Smokers are over one-third more likely to develop migraines compared with nonsmokers. Once smokers are having headaches, using nicotine products lowers their headache threshold. If you need help to quit smoking, try contacting 1-800-QUIT-NOW by phone or online at http://www.smokefree.gov for a free plan and coach.

6. *Watch your diet*

Most people find that skipping meals triggers headaches. Make sure you regularly eat meals throughout the day. Limit caffeinated beverages to no more than two cups or one mug each day. Limit alcohol consumption to a maximum of two drinks per day for adult men and one drink per day for adult women or seniors.

About one in three people can spot a food that triggers headaches. If a food is a trigger, a headache should consistently occur within 12 h of eating it. Keeping a diary of your headaches and the foods you eat can help find your food triggers.

Offer a Limited Supply of Appropriate Interim Medications

Small supplies of interim therapy to treat recurring headaches may include migraine-specific therapies and anti-emetics. Table 9.1 provides recommendations for typical starting doses of acute migraine therapies. Box 9.3 provides an instruction sheet to help explain how patients should use headache therapy, including important distinctions between acute and prevention medications.

Limit using opioids as interim therapy. Providing a small amount of short-acting opioids for recurring primary headaches may encourage repeat visits to secure additional supplies of pain medications. Use the techniques discussed in Chap. 8 for patients requesting inappropriate opioids. Because of limited treatment options during pregnancy, it may be reasonable to provide some pregnant patients with a small amount of opioids for use as rescue medication.

Table 9.1 Interim discharge medications for migraine

Acute migraine therapies	
Patients need to be instructed to regularly use no more than 2 days per week	
Drug	Dose
Excedrin	1–2 tablets; may repeat in 6 h
Naproxen	500 mg; may repeat in 12 h
Sumatriptan (Imitrex)	6 mg injection, 20 mg nasal spray, or 50–100 mg pill; may repeat in 2 h
Rizatriptan (Maxalt)	10 mg tablet; may repeat in 2 h
Zolmitriptan (Zomig)	5 mg nasal spray or tablet; may repeat in 2 h
Eletriptan (Relpax)	40–80 mg tablet; may repeat in 2 h
Almotriptan (Axert)	12.5 mg tablet; may repeat in 2 h
Metoclopramide	10 mg tablet or 20 mg rectal suppository. Dose may be repeated in 6 h, if needed
Prochlorperazine	10 mg tablet or 25 mg rectal suppository. Dose may be repeated in 6 h, if needed
Promethazine	12.5–25 mg rectal suppository
Ondansetron	4–8 mg tablet. Dose may be repeated in 12 h, if needed

Box 9.3 Taking Headache Medications

Headache medications can be divided into two groups: medications you take to treat the headache you have right now and medications to prevent future headaches. Medications you take when you have a headache are called *acute therapies*. Medications to prevent future headaches are called *prevention therapies*.

Acute therapies are used to treat the headache you have when you take them. Examples of over-the-counter acute headache therapies are Excedrin, Tylenol, and aspirin. Don't take more acute medication than recommended by your doctor. Taking acute therapies too often can give you problems with side

(continued)

Box 9.3 (continued)

effects and can actually make your headache worse. People who regularly take any acute therapy acute therapy more than two days each week often develop a worsening of their headaches, called *medication overuse headache.*

Your doctor has prescribed the following acute therapy for you: _____

Take this medicine as follows: _____

Prevention therapies are used by people with frequent problem headaches. Prevention therapies won't help the headache you have today. These therapies are used everyday to help prevent headaches coming over the next several weeks. Most prevention therapies take several weeks to start working. If you have frequent headaches, talk to your doctor about possibly starting a prevention therapy.

Taking Care of Headaches Takes More Than a Pill

When you have headaches, you usually have to do more than just take a pill to make your headaches better. Sticking to a regular schedule for meals and sleeping, eating right, avoiding nicotine, and learning exercises and relaxation skills are just some of the effective techniques you can use to help get your headaches under good control.

It's also important to talk about changes in your treatment with your outpatient doctor. Please call Dr. _____ at _____-_____-_____ to arrange for a follow-up visit within the next 2 weeks.

Identify Important Psychological Comorbidity and Refer Patients for Appropriate Services

Migraine patients who most frequently seek ED treatment for their headaches often have comorbid anxiety or depression [6]. Practical screening tools for anxiety and depression are provided in Table 9.2. Identifying patients with comorbid mood disorders and additionally establishing referrals for their management may be important to minimize excessive ED use for headache management in this group. In many cases, behavioral psychologists can help reduce symptoms of psychological distress and teach important pain management techniques, such as relaxation, biofeedback, and stress management, that have been consistently shown to reduce headache severity and impact. Patients may additionally be referred to useful online resources to get started with relaxation and stress management techniques (Box 9.2).

Table 9.2 Screeners for psychological distress (based on the General Anxiety Disorder-7 [GAD-7] [8] and the Depression in Medically Ill screen [DMI-10] [9] and reprinted with permission from Marcus DA. Chronic pain. A primary care guide to practical management. 2nd ed. New York: Humana Press; 2009)

A. Do you have problems with anxiety?

Choose the one description for each item that best describes *how many days* you have been bothered by each of the following over the past *2 weeks*:

	None Score = 0	Several Score = 1	7 or more Score = 2	Nearly every day Score = 3
Feeling nervous, anxious, or on edge				
Unable to stop worrying				
Worrying too much about different things				
Problems relaxing				
Feeling restless or unable to sit still				
Feeling irritable or easily annoyed				
Being afraid that something awful might happen				

Scoring: Sum scores from each question. A total score 5–9 suggests mild anxiety, while a score ≥ 10 suggests moderate–severe anxiety.

B. Do you have problems with your mood?

Please rate each statement, considering how you have been feeling in the last 2–3 days compared with how you normally feel:

	Not true Score = 0	Slightly true Score = 1	Moderately true Score = 2	Very true Score = 3
I find myself stewing over things.				
I feel more vulnerable than usual.				
I am critical of or hard on myself.				
I feel guilty.				
Nothing seems to cheer me up.				
I feel like I've lost my core or essence.				
I feel depressed.				
I feel less worthwhile.				
I feel hopeless or helpless.				
I feel distant from other people.				

Scoring: Sum scores from each question. A total score ≥9 suggests depression.

Arrange for Headache Follow-up with an Outpatient Provider

A recent study evaluated the impact of insurance status on migraine care in the USA [7]. Researchers determined that patients with no insurance or Medicaid were twice as likely to be treated with no migraine-specific abortive treatment (i.e., triptan or ergotamine) or standard migraine preventive drug than those with private insurance. When analyzed further, a significant contributor to this care discrepancy was the fact that uninsured and Medicaid patients were more likely to receive their migraine care in the ED. A total of 34% of migraine care occurred in the ED for uninsured or Medicaid patients compared with 13% for privately insured patients. These data highlight that the ED can be an important stopgap measure for un- or under-insured headache sufferers, but effective long-term treatment is facilitated by interfacing with regular, outpatient healthcare providers.

Strategies to facilitate successful outpatient follow-up include:

- Providing patients with names and contact information of providers in their area interested in managing chronic headaches.
- Having the discharge nurse contact the patient's doctor to arrange timely follow-up prior to discharge.
- Contacting the patient 24–48 h after discharge to verify that a follow-up appointment was arranged.

Patients can also be provided with a card to complete with their outpatient provider to provide detailed information about medical diagnoses, medications, and recommendations for chronic headache treatment (Box 9.4). This card can provide useful information about treatment options and specific details about reported medication allergies and sensitivities that have been verified by the patient's treating healthcare provider.

Box 9.4 Patient Headache Information Card

When you meet with your doctor, please complete the following card and keep this information in your wallet. Be sure to update as your health and medications change.

Name:_____ Headache diagnosis:_____

Additional medical conditions: _____

_____

Medications allergies or sensitivities (list medication and the reaction that occurs when you take it):_____

_____

What is your current headache treatment:_____

_____

If you come to the emergency department for your usual headaches when your usual medications haven't worked, what alternative medications would your doctor prefer that you receive?_____

_____

Doctor's name, signature, phone number, & date:_____

_____

Summary

- Patients treated in the ED for acute headache have a high rate of return visits. Strategies to reduce inappropriate return visits should be routinely utilized.
- At discharge, patients need clear written information about their headache diagnosis and instructions for managing residual pain or recurring headaches.
- An interim headache-management strategy given to the patient at ED discharge should contain instructions for treating headache-related nausea and pain.
- Post-ED treatment may include limited supplies of an anti-emetic, nonsteroidal anti-inflammatory drug, and triptan.
- Outpatient referral for the management of headache and comorbid psychological distress (e.g., depression and anxiety) can help reduce repeated ED visits.

References

1. Gupta MX, Silberstein SD, Young WB, et al. Less is not more: underutilization of headache medications in a university hospital emergency department. Headache. 2007;47:1125–33.
2. Friedman BW, Hochberg ML, Esses D, et al. Recurrence of primary headache disorders after emergency department discharge: frequency and predictors of poor pain and functional outcomes. Ann Emerg Med. 2008;52:696–704.
3. Friedman BW, Solorzano C, Xia S, et al. Treating headache recurrence after emergency department discharge: a randomized controlled trial of naproxen versus sumatriptan. Ann Emerg Med. 2010;56:7–17.
4. Martins IP, Gouveia RG. More on water and migraine. Cephalalgia. 2007;27:372–4.
5. Spigt MG, Kuijper EC, van Schayck CP, et al. Increasing the daily water intake for the prophylactic treatment of headache: a pilot trial. Eur J Neurol. 2005;12:715–8.
6. Villiani V, Di Stani F, Vanacore N, et al. The "repeater" phenomenon in migraine patients: a clinical and psychometric study. Headache. 2010;50:348–56.
7. Wilper A, Woolhandler S, Himmelstein D, Nardin R. Impact of insurance status on migraine care in the United States: a population-based study. Neurology. 2010;74:1178–83.
8. Spitzer RL, Kroenke K, Williams JW, Löwe B. A brief measure for assessing generalized anxiety disorder. The GAD-7. Arch Intern Med. 2006;166:1092–7.
9. Parker G, Hilton T, Bains J, Hadzi-Pavlovic D. Cognitive-based measures screening for depression in the medically ill: the DMI-10 and the DMI-18. Acta Psychiatr Scand. 2002;105:419–6.

Index

medical emergency, 160, 161
positive biopsy findings, 163
steroid-related complications, 163, 164
stroke, 160
symptoms, 48
Gastric stasis, 84
Glasgow coma scale (GCS), 32–33
Glucocorticoids, 162

H
Headache History Collection Form, 26
Headache recurrence
post-ED follow-up care, 198
pregnancy, 137
Hemicrania continua, 5
Hypertension, 13–15, 34
Hypnic headache
characteristics, 165
diagnosis, 165
ED treatment, 166
features, 165
ICHD-II diagnostic criteria, 5

I
Ice pick headache, 5
Idiopathic intracranial hypertension
characteristics of, 76
increased intracranial pressure, 75, 76
lumbar pressures, 77–78
papilledema, 77
pregnancy, 134
spinal fluid examination, 42
symptoms, 76, 77
treatment, 78
Immediate Postconcussion Assessment and
Cognitive Testing (ImPACT), 59–60
Interim care
ED discharge summary sheet, 198–199
effective strategies, chronic headaches,
199–200
rehydration, 198
return visit, 197
Interim therapy
headache medications
acute therapies, 201–202
pills, 202
prevention therapies, 202
migraine, 201
opioids, 201
Intracranial mass lesion, 55
Ipsilateral headache, 61

Ischemic stroke
cervicocranial arterial dissection, 61
CT scan, 40
migraine and risk of, 72

J
Jolt Accentuation Test, 70

L
Lactation
cluster headache treatment, 150
migraine treatment
analgesics, 149–150
anti-emetics, 149
ED headache treatment, 147, 148
rehydration, 142–143
safety rating system, 141–142
Latent trigger point, 105
Lidocaine, 146
Litigation risk
attitude errors, 187
cognitive errors
context and availability errors, 186
premature closure errors, 185, 186
communication techniques, 184
informed consent, 189–190
recognized treatment method, 189
reducing common errors, 187–189
signal-to-noise error, 186–187
standard of care, 189
Lumbar puncture
adults, normal results, 46
cerebral venous thrombosis, 74
idiopathic intracranial hypertension, 77–78
landmark identification, 42, 43
leaning forward position, 44
patient positioning and needle
placement, 42, 43

M
Magnetic resonance imaging (MRI)
cerebral venous thrombosis, 74
cervicocranial arterial dissection, 61
Chiari malformation, 122
cluster headache, 41–42
colloid cyst, 28
cystic tumor, 55
meningitis, 71
pregnant and nursing patients, 136, 139–141
subdural hemorrhage, 159